CW01513243

Dear Barbara

I Do Hope You Enjoy The Book
And The Journey It Takes You On.

YOU CAN LIVE A BLACK BELT LIFE

THE GIFT OF LIFE DEVELOPMENT

PHIL TOOGOOD

Published by Phil Toogood Coaching

First published by Phil Toogood Coaching 2022
©Phil Toogood 2022
www.philtoogood.com

This book is not intended as a substitute for medical advice. The reader should consult a doctor in matters relating to his/her health and particularly with respect to any symptoms that may require diagnosis or medical attention.

Cover and text design by Barry Lowenhoff
Lowenhoff Design
lowenhoff@gmail.com

Illustrations by Leo Soph Welton
I am Human, Design for change
www.iamhuman-design.co.uk

ISBN 978-1-7396881-3-4

This book is dedicated to my clients who continue to inspire me every day.

CONTENTS

FOREWORD

I have been teaching karate for nearly six decades and I have taught in several countries around the world.

I first met Phil Toogood over twenty years ago when I was working out at my gym. He came over and introduced himself to me. He said he was fascinated by karate but was too old and stiff to take it up after many years of playing other sports.

I had, at the time, been teaching karate for thirty-five years. I could see and feel in those few moments that here was a person who had the potential to become someone quite special once he started to truly believe in himself. For me, life is about setting and achieving goals and, instantly, I knew my goal for him was to take him on a journey from someone who knew nothing about karate to becoming a black belt. I quickly recognised he had a deep desire to succeed so I used that to persuade him to turn up for his first karate lesson.

He went on to become a sensei and lifelong friend.

Phil's motivation for writing this book is to show other people what is possible with the right attitude and to pass on the knowledge, experience and wisdom he obtained on his journey.

Phil's adventure in the dojo was a tough one for many reasons and he has now skilfully used his learning, the trials, the ups and downs and, especially, that magic moment when all your efforts finally come together as a parallel to what many of us have to deal with outside of a dojo in our day-to-day lives. And this is exactly how he now approaches his clients as a very successful life and transformational coach, helping people take their lives to new levels. In this book, he shares the process for success he uses with his clients and the challenges they are struggling with.

You Can Live a Black Belt Life is quite different to other books on the subject of personal growth and discovery because the author uses science to support experiences and emotions and explains how focussing on the power of the mind can literally bring significant changes to our lives.

One of Phil Toogood's most important attributes is his zest for life which is, of course, reflected both in his way of life and within these pages. He has also developed into a first-class karate instructor. He is one of my closest friends and is always there for me when I need his help in my everyday life.

I urge everyone to read this book and I truly believe you can, and will, benefit from living a black belt life.

Sensei Peter T. Heal
Royal Marine served with 40 Commando, Justice of the Peace (JP), International Trader

PREFACE

I was in London having coffee with my friend and fellow coach, Jane Smart. She said, 'I think you should write a book; you have a great story to tell.'

At the time I was designing a life and leadership programme using my adventure into the world of karate as a metaphoric framework. I was carrying out motivational speaking engagements that focussed on mental health at work. I called the presentations 'The gateway to greater mental fitness' and 'The gateway to mind and body mastery'. I found a way of developing the system used in the karate journey, from starting as a white belt, progressing through the grades to become a black belt, as a way of communicating self-development and growth in our everyday lives.

The codes of conduct and the written precepts used in karate, along with the brilliantly clear, clever and inspirational goal-setting process, when unpacked and evaluated, all linked to improving performance. I considered this to be an ingenious system for achievement. So simple, yet hugely stretching and challenging, nonetheless. I truly believed it could become a template that could be applied to work/life success.

Having taken the journey, within martial arts, lasting for twenty years or so I tasked myself with figuring out what drove me and others to embark on this route. How does anyone find the mental strength, develop amazing new skills and above all discover the spiritual element that is crucial to bring about change? I then had my epiphany. I realised that each and every one of us face similar challenges to those that occur in martial arts; overcoming our fears, dealing with self-limitations and constantly battling with our minds and what the world throws at us. All this while trying to find that inner peace and calmness we all crave.

I pieced together the answers, gained from some deep reflection, and studied the fascinating results from the One Word Survey (that follows this preface) and began to design a journey that everyone can experience. An intriguing, exciting, rewarding, potentially life-changing adventure of learning, development and self-discovery, a journey from white belt living to living a black belt life.

I am convinced that each and every one of us has the resources and untapped inner wonders that can help us all to grow as human beings in so many ways. This book outlines a journey of self-development; it will be different for each of you. I sincerely hope you discover something unique and special, personal to only you, that helps to take you to another level of life.

Please trust me when I say, 'You can live a black belt life.'
What is a black belt life?
You are about to discover exactly that!

ONE WORD SURVEY

centred — calm — hard — smart — **positive** — undaunted — no ego — controlled
aware — **mindful** — disciplined — dedicated — strong — committed — masterful
meditative — measured — fluid — confident — has presence — grounded
umble — inwardly strong — **courageous** — flexible — agile — respected
estful — respectful — ambitious — driven — motivated
has humility empowered
unphased — balanced fast — determined
relaxed — precise present — special
glowing — **has belief** trained — **elite**
ole model — inspiring — energetic balanced — healthy
well-being — centred — self-reliant proud — **fulfilled**
precise — sensei — leader — peaceful persistent — **resilient**
wellness — single-minded — gifted resilient — cool — **strong**
humble — sharp — frightening awesome — spirited
evoted — **trained** — smart — clear — grateful — relentless
dedicated — spirited — strong mindset — complete
teacher — learning — self-controlled willpower — **composed**
tough — **purposeful** — giving principled — humble
exceptional — amazing — hardworking skilled — powerful
enerous — consistent — **understanding** **focussed** — controlled
impressive — scary — fierce — accomplished — achiever — winner — peaceful — accurate
self-aware — self-esteem — believing — serious — resolute — fearless — best
extraordinary — spiritual — attention to detail — happy — restrained — motivational

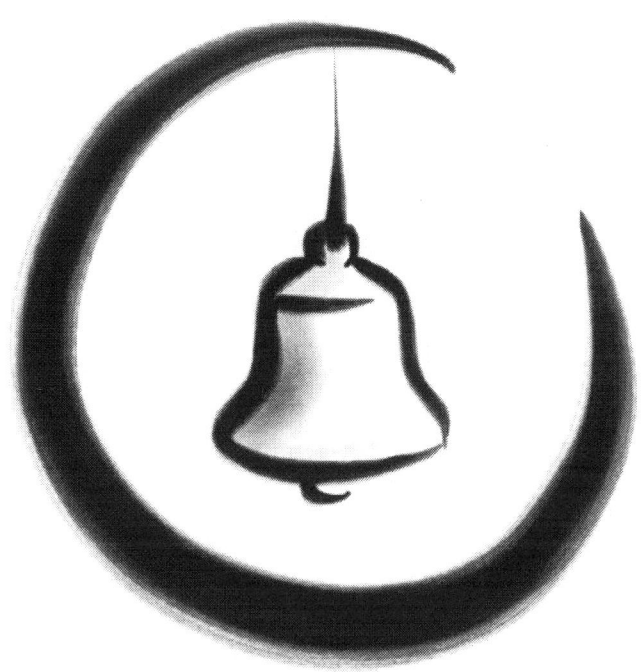

INTRODUCTION

'Our greatest glory is not in never failing, but in rising every time we fail.' ~ CONFUCIUS

When I was forty-one years old, I was at my gym, where I'd been a member for many years, and noticed a guy wearing a beautiful white gi (martial arts uniform). He had a yellow belt wrapped around his waist. Although I'd played amateur sports, predominantly cricket, to a reasonably high level I had always been in awe of martial artists. I have met a few throughout my life and they all seem to have something different, something special about them. I couldn't actually put my finger on it; I can only describe it as a sort of presence. To me, they were not like other people.

I made a point of speaking to the chap in the gi, whose name was Piers, and fired off all sorts of questions which he translated into thinking I wanted to join the club. This was as far from my intention as you could get. It didn't cross my mind for one second. I was just interested in what they did and how they did it. I was not planning to take up karate in my forties.

He moved a little closer and proceeded to tell me the days they trained. I reacted defensively and told him all the reasons why this would be impossible, citing my age (Piers was close to half my age) and the condition of my body after twenty-five years of cricket and fast bowling. I then went into great detail about the state of my back, hips and hamstrings, and further explained how stiff and locked up I was. By this time, he'd stopped listening. He pointed to, what I would politely describe as, an elderly gentleman roughly twenty-five to thirty years my senior, who was doing reps on a nearby sit-up machine, and said, 'Go and speak to Peter, he's the club sensei.'

The next sixty seconds changed my life. It would have been so easy for me not to make that short walk to introduce myself to Sensei Peter. Already there is a lesson learned.

I walked over and the closer I got the more I felt his aura. I paused in front of him and said, 'Piers suggested I introduce myself to you, my name is Phil.'

'So you'd like to join the club?' he said. I launched into the same spiel I had used on Piers as to why I wasn't fit to join. Peter looked at me, his eyes fixed on mine, and said, 'Phil, give me twelve months with you and I will get you doing things you can only dream of.'

The truth is, in response, I felt a rush of emotion – an unusual mixture of adrenaline, excitement, courage and confidence that merged together to give me a strange feeling of power. This all happened in a split second. That one sentence opened up a gateway, that, when I took just one step through it, unleashed me into a new world.

Within a few days, at approximately 7.00 pm, I was staring at the door of the dojo – the room where martial arts is practised, dressed in a white T-shirt and blue and white Adidas tracksuit bottoms. My heart was racing. What lay beyond the door? I was stepping into something I had never experienced before, into the unknown. It would have been so easy to turn around and walk away or retreat upstairs to watch the training session from the viewing gallery.

But I opened the door and walked into a room full of people, all wearing pristine white gis. Sensei Peter was at the far end of the room and acknowledged me with a nod of the head. I had no understanding whatsoever of the ethics and philosophy that underpin this amazing art. Suddenly, Sensei Peter shouted, 'Line up!' There immediately followed a few seconds of brisk activity while people moved around to find their position, filling the air with the strange noise movement of the gi makes. Then there was complete silence. There was literally no sound.

I didn't know what to do, or where to go. It was quickly pointed out to me that everyone was lined up in order of status, with the lowest grade on the left. So, to give you an idea of my grade, my status, when I looked left I was staring at the wall!

This was it. My success on the cricket field, everything I had achieved in my career meant absolutely nothing. I was emotionally stripped naked. Any ego was left on the other side of the dojo door. Standing to my right, with a far greater rank than me, were people half my age. In those few seconds, which seemed like an eternity, several confusing thoughts entered my head. The first one being, *What the hell am I doing here?*

The sensei shouted, *'Yoi!'*, which is Japanese for 'ready' or 'prepare'. A second later everyone was focussed waiting for the next instruction.

Sensei Peter looked at me and said, 'You will have to copy the person to your right to begin with.' I had never before felt so inadequate.

I glanced to the right where everyone was standing in a position of almost robotic concentration. I bent forward slightly so I could see the line of people wearing this wonderful white uniform, all sporting different coloured belts – orange, red, yellow, green, purple, brown. I bent over further so I could see the end of the line where the black belts were standing. I was star-struck by this elite group of people.

Can I make that journey down the line of coloured belts and one day stand at the other side of the dojo? Could I really achieve this? Should I go for it? Why am I doing this? Even though 'the journey' was only 30 feet across the floor it would take years to reach that special place at the far end. A 30-feet journey that takes years to travel. Incredible.

Another instruction blasted out in Japanese and the class reacted in unison to complete a move in military-style precision. That is, with the exception of me. For the next torturous hour, I found myself facing the opposite direction to every other student, time and time again. To say I struggled is an understatement.

Yet again, I asked myself: *Why am I doing this?* The fear of failure, the unknown, rejection, humiliation and criticism started to get into my head. My confidence was shattered, my self-worth was zero and my ego was in danger of preventing me from ever entering that dojo again. *Do I really need to do this at this point in my life? Should I return to face that door again in three days' time?*

I didn't know it then, but I was already on my own private, personal journey of self-discovery and I'm about to share my learning and transformation with you using this unique experience as a metaphor for what each and every one of us go through at some point in our lives. Your trip of a lifetime to self-mastery begins here.

This is not just another self-help book. It is a powerful journey; and it's going to be your journey. Follow the syllabus and you will travel down the line of belts and reach the other end to stand with the black belts in life. I will provide you with the models, tips, tools, skills, guidance; brain training and mind maintenance you need to build your own bulletproof system that will lead you to that magical place dreams are made of, that unique place of self-control and inner peace.

This book is designed to provide you with a deeper knowledge of 'self', of you. It's designed to tap into your inner potential to discover the best version of you. My aim is to teach you new skills and arm you with tools that allow you to press pause, risk assess and perform with confidence in all the arenas of your life. No matter who you are, how old you are or what physical or emotional shape you are in, this book will provide the inspiration you need to change your life. It will motivate you, lift your performance levels and provide the clarity, meaning and purpose to help you alter the course of your life.

In my profession as a life and performance coach, I have worked with many people who have transformed their lives. I have witnessed them having many 'aha' moments, powerful epiphanies that dramatically affected the way they look, feel and deal with life. I have worked with people from all walks of life, including many high performers, who work hard to improve themselves. However, they constantly battle with anxiety, low confidence and damaged self-worth, as well as mental health challenges, such as depression, and well-being issues. I am lucky enough to have been with them when they celebrate their successes, make remarkable changes to their lives, win their inner battles, make career changes, improve relationships, manage stress and transform their mindset to one of peace, progress and positivity.

One of my clients reversed clinically diagnosed depression, in six months, after many years of suffering. After working together for only half a year, he took the same test that had originally confirmed the diagnosis of clinical depression, and the results were astonishing. I observed a transformation taking place in front of my eyes – a straighter back, a more purposeful stride, a natural smile and genuine engagement and laughter. Over time, a new confidence and purpose started to evolve in him. He is the perfect example of what we can achieve if we put our mind to it. The key word here is 'mind'.

Earlier I defined the dojo as a room where martial arts is practised. Translated dojo means 'place of the way'. Traditionally, the dojo is said to take on two aspects. The first, as the training centre and learning ground for martial arts, the second as a place to develop and grow as a person, as a human being. To unlock and develop unseen strengths from untapped potential while overcoming your fears and frailties.

That is 'the place'. So, what is 'the way'?

For me it's almost too special to capture in words. The way is a mystical pathway, a route, a journey, a passage of time dedicated to commitment, change, growth and transformation. If you keep on the way no matter what is thrown at you to send you off course, and continue to follow the path with grit and determination, I promise you will end up in a very special place indeed. This book will show you the way to an awakening, described by the famous American author Deepak Chopra, as the state of being when you are no longer living in a dream world. You awaken to understanding who you really are in a deeper sense; your inner world. You awaken from the inside out.

For me, one of the most beautiful things about this book is that, apart from picking it up and reading it, you do not have to go anywhere or invest in anything new. The answers, the tools, the wisdom to finding the way, exist within you, hence my brand philosophy being INSiDEOUT LIVING. I often describe this as an attitude towards life that transcends our existence producing a more meaningful and fulfilling life.

I eventually came to realise exactly what I had put myself through to become a black belt. From the first meeting with Sensei Peter and walking through the dojo door at, what then seemed like, the ridiculous age of forty-one, to the fears, setbacks, injuries, and mental obstacles I had to face. I came close to giving up many times. I realised this was a journey many of us face every day, not in the dojo, but in life. I now understand what I endured mentally, physically, emotionally, spiritually and scientifically. More importantly, I have unravelled the mystery as to what kept me going from beginning to end, from white belt to black.

In order to better understand how the general public view a black belt in martial arts, I subsequently conducted a survey (the One Word Survey, reproduced at the beginning of this book). I asked people I came in contact with to answer this question: How would you describe a black belt in one word? The results were fascinating. I kept looking at them and realised all of the words on the list can be applied to everyone. We can all become black belts in life. This survey convinced me to write *You Can Live a Black Belt Life.*

I have, therefore, written a book that contains my own personal experiences and subsequent learning, both in and out of the dojo. I use the time spent in the dojo as a parallel of life looking at the physical, mental, emotional and spiritual sides to our being. There are some key messages within these pages, as you will discover, but I must share an important one with you here – *if I can do it, anyone can!*

Human beings are learning machines and I intend to take advantage of this to help you find inner peace, happiness born from experiencing self-acceptance and personal fulfilment. I want to help you to discover new and exciting things about yourself, venturing into unchartered territories of your potential to unleash on the world.

The goal of this book is to take you on a journey of inner self-exploration, an adventure whereby you will be able to enjoy new learning, gain new life-supporting tools, greater confidence and self-worth and convert them into special skills that will enable you to design a new version of your life.

Playwright and Nobel Prize winner, George Bernard Shaw famously said, *'Life is not about finding yourself. Life is about creating yourself.'* I truly believe it's a bit of both as we have so much potential locked away, awaiting discovery. I want you to treat this book as your treasure map to find those hidden gems and, from that point onwards, you can then begin to create something remarkable. The aim of this book is to help you feel alive!

When you open this book, you will be entering a special and sacred gateway into the dojo of life. It will show you how to transform your life, through eight steps of transition, corresponding to the belts in karate, from white to black, and guide you to places you didn't know existed within you. Along the way, you will be challenged and stretched. You will ask yourself many questions. I promise it will be *you* that finds the answers.

This book is for anyone who has ever suffered with low confidence, poor self-esteem and a genuine lack of self-worth. It is for all those who suffer from negative, demotivating and demeaning self-talk, regularly overthinking situations and anyone who finds it difficult to control and manage their emotions. It's for all of you who have reached a crossroads or dead end in your life and are looking for a compass to navigate you to somewhere new. It's for people who find themselves living a life of comparison and excuses, always looking outwards at how well others are doing and then creating judgements and justifications that keep the fire of jealousy burning within.

It's for anyone who spends their time consciously suffering feelings of guilt and regret about their past and/or is in a constant state of worry and anxiety about the future. It's also for people who live with the pain of fear. Fear of the unknown, rejection and failure.

And finally, this book is for everyone who wants to take their life to another level no matter where they start from. It's for high performers who want to challenge themselves to see if they can achieve even greater heights, as well as those just starting out in their chosen career.

I list these issues because I have faced them all myself throughout my life. After years of reflection, research and reinvention, believe me when I say that the tips, tools and techniques I'm going to share with you, changed my life for the better. I have no doubt they will change yours, too.

However, I must be clear from the outset that to create a change in direction, re-engineer your life and achieve the results you are hoping to obtain, you will be stretched and pushed outside of your personal comfort zone into a world of new learning and development. Change requires hard work!

I have designed this book so that you don't actually need to buy a gi, join a club, get licensed and go through years of physical and mental training in martial arts. All you have to do is immerse yourself in this book as if it was your own unique and private dojo and then simply follow the way.

Each chapter represents a different coloured belt, the same as in karate. The journey from white to black is hugely significant, it's a process, just as it is in the dojo. Move through each chapter and gain your belts. Complete the drills, use the tools, create new habits and adhere to the six pillars of the way and you too can live a black belt life.

This book will help you become part of a unique community of people, who all started at exactly the same place and worked their way through a specific journey of tests and challenges metaphorically taking them from living a white belt life to living a black belt life. They learned how to operate within a specific culture that teaches you first and foremost to believe that anything is possible. I want you to realise this from the outset – you can achieve anything. I want you to stretch and challenge yourself. To attempt things, you'd not just thought about but dreamt about.

I truly believe this book will guide you to wonderful destinations, unlocking magnificent and mystical treasures along the way. All you need to do is open up, commit to the process and remember the words of my sensei, *'Give me twelve months with you and I'll get you doing things you could only dream of.'* Treat this book as your sensei, your dojo, your place of the way and you, too, can live a black belt life.

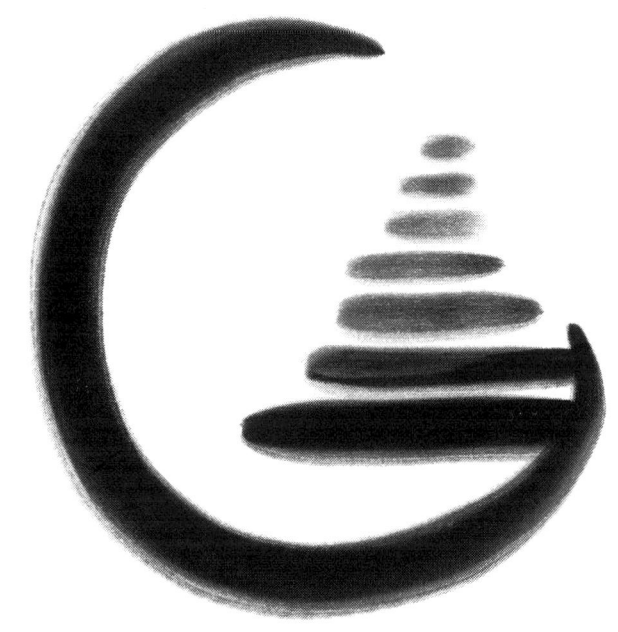

CHAPTER 1
WHITE BELT
Attitude is Everything

'The unexamined life is not worth living.' ~ SOCRATES

The preceding quote by Socrates defines beautifully the process we are about to engage in. We live in two worlds; an outside world that we have little control over and a world inside of us that we can learn to control. So, in the words of Socrates, we begin by examining your life, from the inside out, to see what potential, performance and progress we can unlock. The white belt syllabus provides an understanding of the philosophy and underpinning precepts for this incredible journey ahead. It also encapsulates the message that will continue throughout your journey and support your first few steps on the way to achieving your first grade.

Much of what we achieve in life starts with the belief that we all possess treasures within us that sometimes simply need uncovering or discovering. So many people are walking around with incredible wonders within them that they are yet to unlock and understand. Therefore, to begin our white belt training, I would like to share a story with you, as told by the iconic motivational speaker and hugely successful author Jack Canfield. When I heard it, I thought what an incredibly clever use of a historical story as a metaphor for life, and it really struck a chord with me. As you read it, and throughout this whole book, please keep in mind the white belt mantra — 'attitude is everything'.

It's not a verbatim transcript but somewhere close.

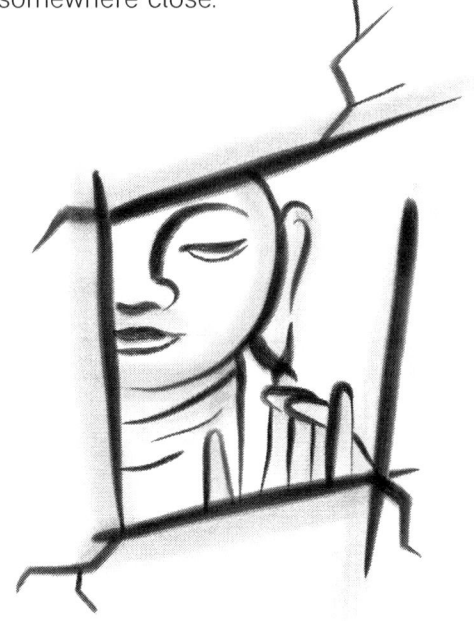

In a Bangkok temple there sits a 10-feet tall, 5½ ton, solid gold Buddha. It is believed to have been made around the 13th or 14th century.

The Burmese invaded Thailand, then Siam, in 1767. They were renowned for taking gold statues and melting them down, as well as cutting off the heads of others. The Siamese monks found out about the planned invasion and set out to completely cover the Buddha statue with a clay-type substance to protect it from the looters.

Legend has it that, regrettably, all the monks were slaughtered, leaving the giant golden Buddha a secret until 1957, when a group of monks from a monastery had to relocate the clay Buddha from their temple to a new location. The monastery was to be moved to make room for the development of a highway through Bangkok. When the crane began to lift the huge figure, the weight of it was so tremendous that it began to crack. Then the rain began to fall. The head monk, who was concerned about damage to the sacred Buddha, decided to lower the statue back to the ground and cover it with a large canvas tarpaulin to protect it from the rain.

Later on, the head monk went to check on the Buddha. He shone his flashlight under the cover to see if the Buddha was staying dry. As the light reached the crack, he noticed a little gleam shining back and thought it strange. As he took a closer look at this gleam of light, he wondered if there might be something underneath the clay. He went to fetch a chisel and hammer from the monastery and began to chip away at the clay. As he knocked off chunks of clay, the little glow grew brighter and brighter, and many hours later the monk stood face to face with this astonishing solid gold Buddha.

Jack explains the moral behind this story is that it demonstrates perfectly how, in life, many of us cover up the wonders within. The wonders I, personally, refer to are self-confidence, self-belief, self-esteem and self-love, as well as the wisdom, resilience and skillsets we gain through successes and failures that we can pass on to others. Over time, life's challenges and our way of thinking take their toll. Regret, guilt, anger, anxiety, fears, sadness and worse form a personal clay covering. Metaphorically speaking, this thick, heavy outer layer restricts us from being able to express ourselves and continually develops to a level whereby we are unable to demonstrate our skills and talents to the world.

The statistics in relation to self-confidence and self-belief are horrendous. Dr Joe Rubino, the CEO of The Center for Personal Reinvention, reports that 85% of people suffer with some kind of low self-esteem. It doesn't have to be this way.

In this white belt chapter, you will begin to peel back that covering and discover the wonders each of you holds within. Yes, in truth, it will be challenging, but just imagine how the monk felt when he came face to face with the 10-feet tall, solid gold Buddha. Now imagine feeling the same way about your own amazing discoveries, when you unearth tools and life skills that will prove to be life-changing and transformational.

The white belt syllabus is the beginning of something magnificent. Life in the dojo ensures you are pushed, stretched, tested and challenged. The process helps you to deal with so many of life's inner confrontations and fears that haunt us like innate demons, such as lack of confidence, self-belief and destructive self-talk. It also opens up a world of well-being and self-management.

Entering the dojo for the first time is an incredibly daunting prospect; it feels like entering a sacred temple. It was so different to anything I'd personally experienced before. There is a unique atmosphere within it, an unexplained aura. It feels special but intimidating at the same time. A squash court, sports hall or an aerobics studio, all of which are places to train, learn and develop, can also become this mystical temple, creating a spiritual place of self-improvement. In my experience, football and cricket changing rooms possess a wonderful, united feeling of togetherness; an energy you can embrace and tap into. However, the dojo has something quite unique about it – to the point where it feels almost other-worldly.

The dojo also teaches collaboration, a universal and genuine respect, appreciation and realisation of other people's endeavours, resources and personal achievements, and to recognise that others have their own mountains to climb.

In Japanese 're' means 'bow' and, although it is a simple act, it is treated with the utmost importance. It is a sign of respect and humility to the place of the way and students within it. Students of karate also bow when they meet outside of the dojo especially when they see their sensei (teacher). They always respect him/her with 're' but a softer version than in the dojo. Wherever they meet, they always acknowledge each other with a nod of the head.

It is said that bowing when entering the dojo enables you to leave all your problems at the door, helping you to focus solely on your martial art. It's sometimes referred to as 'emptying your cup' and goes back to a conversation that famously took place a long time ago between a scholar named Tokusan and a Zen master named Ryutan. One of the versions of the story goes like this:

There was once a wise Zen master. People travelled miles to seek his help and wisdom. The Zen master would teach them and show them the way to true enlightenment and wisdom in life. On one particular day, a scholar visited the master seeking advice. The scholar approached the master and explained, 'I have come to ask you to teach me about Zen.'

A few minutes into their conversation, it was clear the scholar was convinced of his own views, opinions and knowledge. He interrupted the master continuously with his own stories and failed to listen and be attentive to what the master had to say and teach.

The master calmly suggested that they should have a cup of tea together. The master, with complete confidence, poured his guest a cup. The cup was filled. To the guest's surprise, the master kept pouring tea until the cup overflowed onto the table.

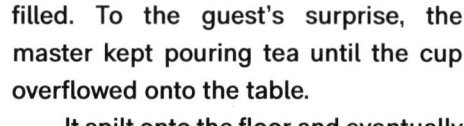

It spilt onto the floor and eventually onto the scholar's jacket. The scholar was astonished and yelled, 'Stop! The cup is full already. Can't you see?'

With a smile, the Zen master replied, 'Empty your cup.' He added that the scholar was just like that cup, full of ideas and convictions, so much so that nothing more can be absorbed, and he advised him to come back with an empty cup!

To help you pass this white belt chapter I would like you to adopt the same approach as the 'Empty Your Cup' story. Bowing is about compassion, feeling and care. It symbolises humility, as there will always be fellow students with more knowledge, experience and skills than you. This humble attitude is such an important trait to have in life as it keeps your ego in check and directs you to think of others.

From this point forwards this book will become your own dojo — your place of the way. Step outside of your day-to-day experiences, allow your mind to find the secrets, discover the wonders within and, ultimately, find the way. When you empty your cup, open the book and bow, you will arrive at the gateway to a new way of living, with a different prospect of what the future might hold. Bow also when you leave, when you close the book.

A simple nod or bow as you open and close the book is all that is required. I ask that you trust me on this and try to embrace this practice before you judge it. As you work through the chapters ahead, it will all make sense.

There are many rules associated with the place of the way but we will be adhering to just a few:

- Respect the book when entering and leaving it. Practise bowing as you open and close the book.
- Keep an open mind (empty your cup) to learning and development. In time, you will develop an inner sensei to listen to and help you on your journey of transformation.
- Clarity and repetition are key to success. This is how to develop new habits that will change your life.
- Practice makes perfect. Throughout the way, the transition to transformation, we must cultivate a 'practice makes perfect' mindset. If you aim for perfection, you will hit outstanding along the way.

As I said in the introduction, in karate, there is a hierarchy of skills and experience set out by the way we line up in the dojo. From left to right, you can see the gradings get higher so all those in the line can look right to see a row of beautifully pressed, white gis and a variety of coloured belts leading up to the black belts on the far right. I would stand in line, on the far left, wondering if I could make that journey across the floor. Now I realise this line of students and coloured belts represented the way, a unique and special pathway to a different life.

It is said that the ultimate goal for many of us is inner peace and a sense of spiritual freedom, to reach a point where there is no need to forgive any longer as we have eliminated all blame from our soul. We have removed all judgement, guilt and anger. We are free from stress and acknowledge and embrace life as it is. What a beautiful place to be.

If you think of life as the seasons of the year, it highlights the importance of living for the moment: 0–20 is your spring, 20–40 is your summer, 40–60 is your autumn and 60–80, and hopefully beyond, is your winter. Don't get to the winter of your life wishing you had attempted or achieved more. At the very least, I want you to be able to say, I had a go and did my best.

As with many things in life – preparation is key. I'm sure you've heard the saying 'fail to prepare, prepare to fail'. In the warm-up before every karate training session, we stretch to help our flexibility. During this process we take our muscles outside the normal 'safe zone'. This is what I intend to do with your mindset, your personal psychology. Stretching is a key element to gaining muscle. Stretching gives the muscle more room to expand. The mind is like a muscle; it also needs stretching. I'm going to stretch your thinking and expand the scope of your mind.

Bruce Lee said, *'Preparation for tomorrow is hard work today.'* Throughout your journey, we will work on applications to develop crucial tools for life, enabling you to uncover motivation and inspiration and access your A-game when you need it.

As a part of the white belt training I would like to introduce you to *Mokuso,* karate's version of meditation. *Mokuso* translated means 'silent thought'. It is carried out before every training session as an essential part of the preparation process to clear the mind and again at the end to reflect on what you have achieved during the session.

The practice of *Mokuso* in the dojo prepares you to let go of the troubles of the day, be mindful of the present moment, gauge your state of mind but also focus on what you want to achieve in the session ahead. It's said to take you back to the state of a newborn child, no fear, no stress and no pain. Nothing else exists other than 'the now'. In karate, mindfulness is introduced to you from the very beginning.

Before each training session begins the sensei calls out *'Mokuso'.* Students then kneel in a special position called *seiza,* which originates from a Buddhist posture that is said to be a conduit to one's self-development. For just a few minutes, *Mokuso* removes mental obstacles and prepares your mind for the laser-type focus, concentration and awareness that's needed in karate, but it also melts away any ego that may be present allowing the mind to achieve a balanced state. At the end of the class, *Mokuso* is called again but this time to wind down and reflect. It's such a beautiful and amazing experience.

Most humans spend most of their time psychologically living in the past or in the future. This avoidance of being 'in the moment' can lead to many mental health-related issues, such as guilt, regret, frustration, disappointment, anxiety and depression.

Now, can you begin to imagine incorporating *Mokuso* into your daily routine? Spending a few moments of quietness, centring yourself into the present moment while focussing on the day ahead. And then, at the end of the day, returning to the dojo of your mind to reflect on what's occurred, what you have learnt, given or gained, as a person that day. It doesn't need to be done in a dark and silent room. Once you become skilled you can do this in a busy and crowded place such as on a train or walking from your place of work.

Daily meditation has been described as the perfect passive activity for the health of a human being. We will deep dive into mindfulness and meditation as we travel through the higher grades, as these are essential elements to accessing your potential for self-mastery.

I would like to suggest that from now on when you pick up this book, before you begin to read, you spend one minute or so working on shutting down the outer world, clearing some space by 'emptying your cup'. Acknowledge any thoughts that come into your mind and let them pass without judgement. This short time will help you to focus on the present moment, removing past and future thinking, bringing you into the true and purest moment in your life. How amazing is that? It will take practice and discipline, as will all the exercises in this book.

In the world of martial arts, our learning begins with stance and balance. This is worked on from the start. We are given drills to help with balance and we work on our stance, posture, weight distribution, head and arm positions. In this book, stance is not about our standing position, stance also means you have a strong belief in something. It's about our attitude, our mindset and how we approach opportunities for new learning. We are searching first for understanding – then comes constant finessing and perfecting new ways and techniques, always progressing and developing.

One of the first things I learnt was repetition becomes an embedded habit. But you must understand what you are doing and why you are doing it in the first place. In the dojo we practise the same move thousands of times so it becomes set in our muscle memory and embedded into our brain. The move becomes a subconscious action, an automatic response.

We are all creatures of habit. This works to our advantage in an amazing way, but remember not all habits are good and we will cover the science behind this as we move across the dojo and through the grades.

In karate, we aim for perfection but never reach it. One of my favourite principles is that when we do a move the next time we must try and execute it a little better. This develops a mindset of continuous improvement and the energy to keep moving forwards, always looking to raise standards. This is a key learning moment in the process. We are taught to follow certain rules. All these rules must be adhered to as part of our journey through the belt gradings. I want to share these rules, or precepts, with you.

To provide you with a little background, Karate, or 'kara-te', translated means 'empty hand' and in this case, no weapons. The origins sprang from a time in history around 500 years ago within an archipelago made up of 161 islands, now named Okinawa, then called the Ryukyu Kingdom, when an invasion resulted in the banning of weapons. This forced the islanders to develop a form of unarmed combat using various techniques to evade, strike, block and throw their attackers.

Okinawa was also the birthplace of Gichin Funakoshi, the founder of modern karate who devised its twenty precepts. This is the style I learnt and still teach today.

'It is important that karate can be practised by the young and the old, men and women alike. That is, since there is no need for a special training place, equipment, or an opponent, a flexibility in training is provided such that the physically and spiritually weak individual can develop his body and mind so gradually and naturally that he himself may not realise his own great progress.' ~ MASTER FUNAKOSHI

The Twenty Precepts – Words of Wisdom to Live by

1. Karate begins with courtesy and ends with courtesy.
2. There is no first attack in karate.
3. Karate is an aid to justice.
4. First control yourself before attempting to control others.
5. Spirit first, technique second.
6. Always be ready to release your mind.
7. Accidents arise from negligence.
8. Do not think that karate training is only in the dojo.
9. It will take your entire life to learn karate; there is no limit.
10. Put your everyday living into karate and you will find myo (subtle secrets).
11. Karate is like boiling water – if you do not heat it constantly, it will cool.
12. Do not think that you have to win, think rather that you do not have to lose.
13. Victory depends on your ability to distinguish vulnerable points from invulnerable ones.
14. The battle is according to how you move, guarded and unguarded (move according to your opponent).
15. Think of your hands and feet as swords.
16. When you leave home, think that you have numerous opponents waiting for you. It is your behaviour that invites trouble from them.
17. Beginners must master low stance and posture; natural body positions are for the advanced.
18. Practising a kata (Japanese for 'form' – a choreographed set of martial arts movements that mimics defensive blocks, attacks and combinations) is one thing, engaging in a real fight is another.
19. Do not forget to correctly apply strength and weakness of power, stretching and contraction of the body and slowness and speed of techniques.
20. Always think and devise ways to live the precepts every day.

Although there are twenty precepts, for me, there is one that is particularly important – precept number 5 – *Spirit first, technique second.* So, for the white belt syllabus, we are going to focus on this precept. I ask that you keep these words in mind as you work your way through this section of the book.

What does this mean? It means that although skillsets are crucial to achieving success, it's the spirit, attitude and what goes on in the mind that will drive you to achieve your goals and more. I often refer to this quote by Lou Holtz, a successful and well-respected former American football coach: *'Ability is what you're capable of doing. Motivation determines what you do. Attitude determines how well you do it.'*

Although every journey will be unique to the individual, the insights you are about to explore will have a dramatic effect on you as a human being. Remember – attitude is everything.

To help you, I am now going to introduce you to my model of the six pillars of the way, the same six pillars I use with every client I coach. If you apply them to your life and goals, and adhere to them strictly, success is guaranteed. You will receive greater clarity as to why the six pillars are the template to success as you travel down the line of belts.

The Six Pillars of the Way:

1. Honesty
2. Trust
3. Commitment
4. Discipline
5. Perseverance
6. Accountability

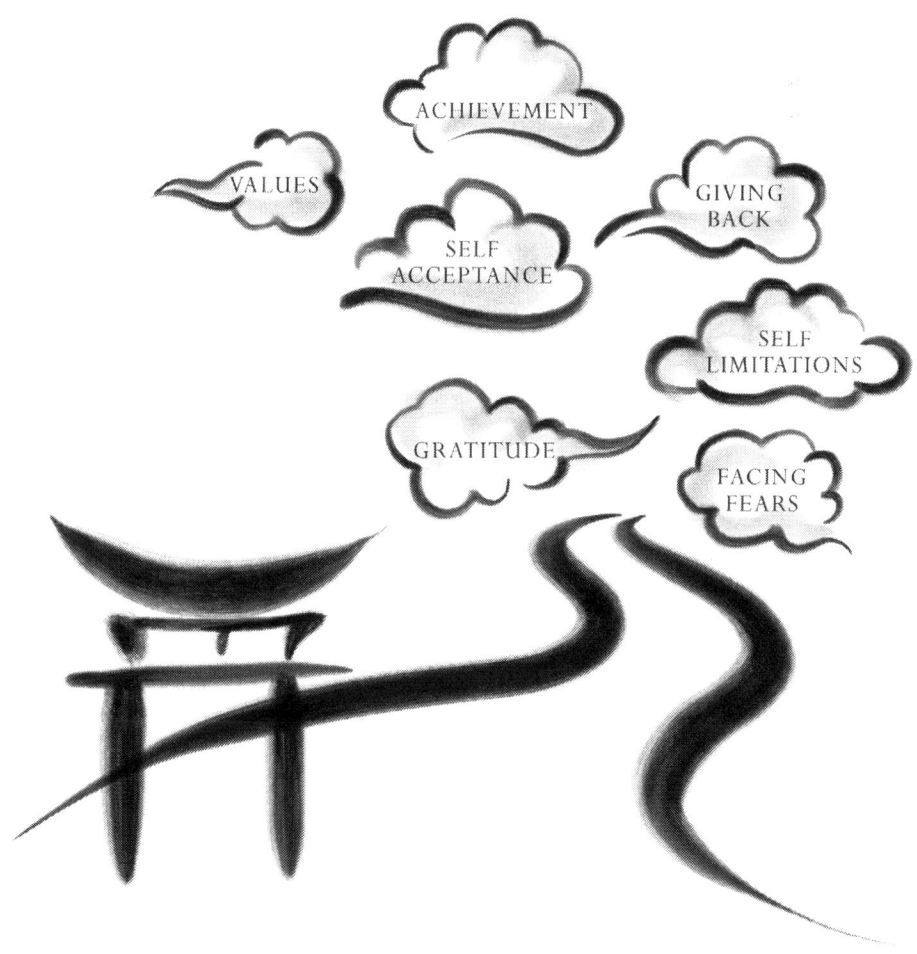

1. HONESTY

This first principle relates to both our inner and outer honesty. Looking at ourselves in the mirror and asking a few questions to judge our reaction. Without honesty from the start there will be no development. How can you measure progress and success without a starting point? It's impossible. The starting point in any self-growth is honesty.

My brother-in-law, Stuart Slater, was a well-recognised and successful professional footballer. I acted as his manager/agent for a short while. During this time, I brokered a record purchase with a premier league club for him to join them. This became the second time he was a record club signing. The manager at the time, John Lyall, was well-respected and was great friends with Sir Alex Ferguson who described him as 'a man of integrity'. It was such an interesting and exciting experience, especially being a football fanatic.

While representing Stuart, once the deal was done and he'd started playing for the club, I was backwards and forwards to meetings with the manager and the assistant manager attempting to get more add-ons to his contract. I was trying to negotiate extras such as a company car and various incentivised bonuses.

Mr Lyall never once refused to see me – he was such a gentleman. One day I was sitting in his office and asked his thoughts on another cash-fuelled performance incentive, this time in the form of a goal bonus. I thought the money would be an incentive for Stuart to become a little greedier with the ball in and around the penalty area, and more clinical in front of goal. That was my thinking anyway.

This great man stood up and spoke. 'OK,' he said. 'I like the idea, but this is how it's going to work…before we hand out yet another giveaway I would like you to consider this as a proposition. If he scores twelve goals before Christmas, I'll make sure he gets a well-rewarded goal bonus. But only after he's netted twelve goals and not before.'

He went on to say, 'These superstars need to take a look at themselves from time to time and ask a few questions. They need to look in the mirror and ask the person staring back at them, "Are you putting in the effort? Are you totally committed?" And be honest about what their reflection is saying.'

I've never forgotten this, it was a great lesson for me from a hugely successful, well-thought-of man who reached the top of his profession. Look in the mirror and be honest with who you are, where you are and where you would like to go.

Therefore, part of the white belt syllabus is to read the following poem by Peter Wimbrow Senior – 'The Man in the Glass'. I first discovered this poem when I read in the press that the England rugby defence coach, Paul Gustard, recited it to the players before the historic match against Australia that took them to their first ever series win in Australia in 2016. It reminded me of what John Lyall had said about Stuart but also had a profound effect on my life in terms of how I looked at myself. It was definitely liberating and ultimately life-changing. So, the drill is to read this poem repeatedly, then reflect on it and on how it made you feel.

THE MAN IN THE GLASS

When you get what you want in your struggle for self
And the world makes you king for a day
Just go to the mirror and look at yourself
And see what that man has to say.
For it isn't your father, or mother, or wife
Whose judgement upon you must pass
The fellow whose verdict counts most in your life
Is the one staring back from the glass.
He's the fellow to please – never mind all the rest
For he's with you, clear to the end
And you've passed your most difficult, dangerous test
If the man in the glass is your friend.
You may fool the whole world down the pathway of years
And get pats on the back as you pass
But your final reward will be heartache and tears
If you've cheated the man in the glass.

Now read it again and perhaps have it as a go-to when you're in need of inspiration or self-reflection.

I want to acknowledge not only the talent of the poet Peter Wimbrow Senior but his attitude towards life, too. When researching permission to use his poem in this book I discovered a website created by Peter's children. It tells how 'The Man in the Glass' as it's commonly known now, was in fact originally written as 'The Guy in the Glass' with a few subtle differences throughout the text. The website says:

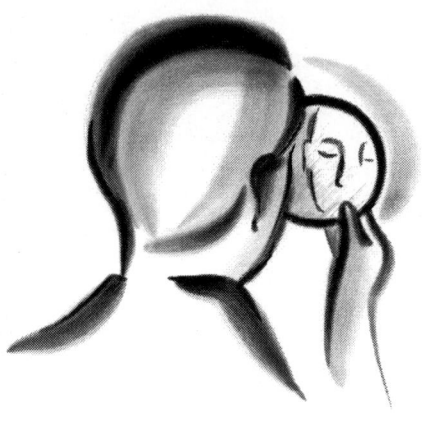

'Our father, Peter 'Dale' Wimbrow Sr. wrote the poem 'The Guy in the Glass' in 1934. It was published in the American magazine at that time and the copyright was assigned to our father. The poem has also become known, incorrectly, as 'The Man in the Glass' or sometimes, 'The Man in the Mirror', but the thought is the same, the message clear...' you can fool the whole world down the pathway of years, but you can't fool the guy staring back from the glass'. Since he wrote the poem in 1934 and it was published, it has taken on a life of its own and is usually seen as anonymous. Sadly, some people have even taken to putting their name on it as their own creation. It escapes us as to why someone would falsely take credit for a poem about being honest with yourself. We are immensely proud of his work and welcome any and all dialogue from interested parties. Our hope here is just to set the record straight and to provide the poem as it was actually written for any and all to use as our father's gift to the world. Our father was the most gifted and caring person we ever knew...he would have wanted his work to be a gift and so do we. All we ask is that you properly credit him somewhere in your publication as the author.'

What an incredibly selfless and generous approach his children have taken to honouring their father's work. Clearly Peter's values and beliefs are shared by his family.

So, in honour of Peter Wimbrow Senior and his children, I wanted to share the original version of the poem with you. Although we will refer back to 'The Man in the Glass' throughout the book, please take a moment to read Peter's original work.

THE GUY IN THE GLASS
by Peter 'Dale' Wimbrow, (c) 1934

When you get what you want in your struggle for self,
And the world makes you king for a day,
Then go to the mirror and look at yourself,
And see what that guy has to say.

For it isn't your father, or mother, or wife,
Who judgement upon you must pass.
The feller whose verdict counts most in your life
Is the guy staring back from the glass.

He's the feller to please, never mind all the rest,
For he's with you clear up to the end,
And you've passed your most dangerous, difficult test
If the guy in the glass is your friend.

You may be like Jack Horner and 'chisel' a plum,
And think you're a wonderful guy,
But the man in the glass says you're only a bum
If you can't look him straight in the eye.

You can fool the whole world down the pathway of years,
And get pats on the back as you pass,
But your final reward will be heartaches and tears
If you've cheated the guy in the glass.

On that note, let's move on to our next pillar – trust.

2. TRUST

Trust is initially about trusting yourself, backing, believing, and having faith in yourself. Open yourself up as a receiver of new learning, bet on your success and believe in yourself. We give ourselves such a hard time. Why is this? Vincent Van Gogh said, *'If you hear a voice within you say, "you cannot paint" then by all means paint, and that voice will be silenced.'*

The trust element of the way is also about trusting the process, believing in the journey and the underpinning messages you will discover but, before anything, please trust yourself. As an orange belt you will acquire tools that will bolster your self-confidence. The more wonders you unearth the greater self-belief and confidence you will gain. As Ralph Waldo Emerson said, 'Self-trust is the first secret of success.'

Trust is the key to success of any team also. This is always a challenge as building trust takes time and effort, it takes success and failure, respect, empathy and total commitment to each other. I am fortunate enough to have been part of a team and to lead teams that were solidly underpinned with trust. It was a wonderful feeling knowing there was this strong sense of respect and honour for each other. Trust is such a difficult thing to find and maintain but it all begins with trusting yourself first. It must start from the inside out before the outside in. Without belief in ourselves we have no goals.

3. COMMITMENT

All six elements of the six pillars of the way require a strong and focussed mindset. Commitment is about showing up and, more importantly, how you show up. Commitment, in this case, is a psychological agreement to the journey; the way.

It is said in karate that you do not get to black belt, you *become* a black belt, and it is the time practising outside the dojo that's most important. I trained two to three times each week but practised every day. I became committed to the process with my mind, body and soul. I created a new way of life, I introduced new habits that would take me to my goal.

When I trained in the dojo, I was surrounded by commitment. I could sense and feel it all around me in the space, and with this sense of commitment, physical, mental and spiritual development seemed to occur naturally.

Sir Bradley Wiggins, arguably one of the greatest cyclists who ever lived, trained on Christmas Day. He did an eighty-six-mile ride one year; his philosophy was that it gave him the edge as none of his competitors would be doing the same. You have to respect and admire that mindset, that determination to give you the upper hand.

I'm not saying that we all have to be like Sir Bradley Wiggins, but he is an example of how far we can take our mind, body and soul – our commitment. There is a wonderful parable, recounted below, that is a perfect illustration of commitment.

THE CHINESE BAMBOO TREE

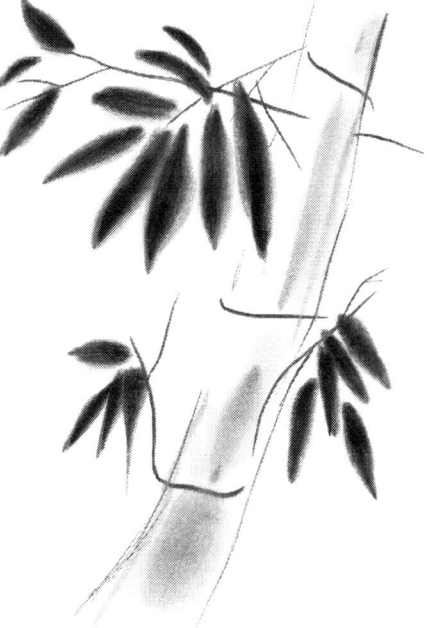

Growing a Chinese bamboo tree requires real trust and commitment. You need to plant that first seed, a seed which, like any other plant, needs constant nurturing.

However, by the end of year one there are no visible signs of activity.

At the end of year two, again, no sign of any growth above the soil.

Years three and four, still nothing.

It's enough to test the patience of any gardener, it becomes easy to question yourself, to wonder if your efforts, care and nurture, will ever pay off. You question whether any of it has worked.

Then comes year five, and...

You don't just see growth, but you see explosive growth at a rate you couldn't have comprehended before! In a six-week period, the Chinese bamboo tree grows to a staggering 90 feet tall – the tree has even been measured to grow 122cm (48 inches) in a twenty-four-hour period.

What an incredible feat of nature!

I use this parable as a metaphor for everything in this book I have experienced myself. I worked hard in the dojo and at various things in my life, especially personal development. Then, when you least expect it – BOOM – you experience this incredible feeling, it's like a rush or an injection of self-confidence, an awakening, that, at times, can be almost overwhelming. Bob Proctor, philosopher and self-help author, describes it as, 'moving up onto another frequency'. I have experienced this many times. I have to say it's an amazing feeling when it all comes together, something just clicks.

The work I did to get there was the root system of the bamboo tree. It developed through commitment, repetition and trust in the process. When working to become an orange belt, we will create a strong platform from which to harness your energy, skills and potential, ready to unleash them when the time is right. The incredible motivational speaker Tony Robbins, whom I hugely admire, said: 'The only limit to your impact is your imagination and commitment.'

4. DISCIPLINE

Discipline can be described as showing up when you least feel like it. Discipline is the glue that sticks all six pillars together. Nothing works without discipline. You can be honest and committed in your mind but without doing the drills, practising new routines and creating new rituals on time, every time, and constantly pushing outside of your comfort zone you will never create new life-changing habits in your life. Without applying discipline how do we create change? The truth is, it's impossible to create change without it.

Aristotle said, 'The whole is greater than the sum of its parts.' Discipline for me creates this outcome. It fuses the six pillars together which produces the energy and power. I think Jim Rohn, another famous author and motivational god summed up discipline perfectly when he said, 'Discipline is the bridge between goals and accomplishment.' I do not believe that it could be defined more accurately.

There is a Chinese proverb by Chinese philosopher and reformer, Confucius, that goes like this:

I hear I forget
I see I remember
I do I understand.

I reference this regularly in my coaching practice. It's the 'doing' that's the tough part but we must embrace it and focus on the benefits and what we are achieving rather than what we are sacrificing. When focussing on achievement and discipline, the word 'sacrifice' can be construed as negative, rather than positive. It emphasises what you are giving up rather then what you are gaining. Do people who are goal orientated and possess a clear purpose focus on what they are sacrificing? No, they don't. The word 'sacrifice' is not in their vocabulary. Their mindset is set to what they are gaining not what they are giving up or losing. These people follow things through. Discipline is following things through. To create any sort of change, discipline is needed more than any other value.

The Special Forces say the difference between them and the rest is mental discipline. Many other elite military regiments are as skilled and physically fit as the Special Forces, the major difference is mental strength and discipline.

5. PERSEVERANCE

You must adhere to the principle 'practice makes perfect' as that's how your actions become embedded into a specific part of your brain so they become automatic. We will touch on the science relating to this as you move up through the grades.

In karate you must quickly adapt to a particular mindset of 'repetition breeds perfection'. Basically, this translates into accepting you're always and forever seeking the means to improve. Every move, every kick, every block and every punch can always be honed, polished and executed a little better. The journey to success, to perfection, is driven by perseverance.

Perseverance brings with it a strength of mind. It teaches you that correction is simply feedback and learning not criticism. Failure is exactly the same. I wouldn't be being true to myself if I didn't share with you that, at times, while learning karate, it was a real struggle. On occasion, I found it torturous to take the shakes of the head from the senseis, a tweaking here and a correction there, a feeling of never getting it quite right. However, I persevered and kept returning for more until one day my mindset changed to 'bring it on' and 'watch me'. I want more attention and instruction. I want to learn more. It just suddenly became normal. I do believe that ego had a part to play as this gets in the way of progress for many of us.

In short, I entered the dojo with a fixed mindset and transitioned into a person with a growth mindset. In her book, *Mindset: The New Psychology of Success*, Dr Carol Dweck writes *'You have a choice...mindsets are beliefs. They're powerful beliefs but just something in your mind and you can change your mind'.* This is a point worth remembering. We can make choices as to how we think and behave. It's within our control. It's inner world stuff.

Dr Dweck talks about fixed mindset people who want to succeed, they try to prove themselves but are incredibly sensitive about being wrong or making mistakes. Whereby a growth mindset person approaches mistakes and failure as learning and, therefore, constantly puts themselves out there to be stretched and challenged. She continues to say growth mindset students look at a teacher as a resource for learning. I think that is a brilliant way to look at life. *'People with a growth mindset don't just seek challenge, they thrive on it',* she says. We change our mindset, and setting powerful goals forces you into a growth mindset state.

This change in mindset helped mould my teaching and coaching methodology as an instructor, particularly with juniors. Training has to be fun first as this accelerates learning and development and, although we still stick to the strict codes of the martial art, I now adopt an approach to teaching that offers a more equal balance between instructing, coaching and encouraging a student. This method has proved to be hugely successful with my younger students. Basically, once in the dojo, I help to engineer their mindset. To this day, it makes me smile when I offer a class of juniors the opportunity to demonstrate their skills, whatever their grade, and someone pops their hand up and says, 'I will, sensei.' I think to myself: *You will go a long way.*

Perseverance is a powerful quality and an integral element of continuous improvement. We are all capable of becoming a better leader, an improved listener, more compassionate, a better husband, wife, parent, teacher, brother, sister, child and so on. Think of the people in your life that might benefit from your own personal growth. It's not a smooth ride, though. As Les Brown, another brilliant American author and motivational speaker says, '...*if it was easy, we'd all be smart, fit and rich'*!

To create change you must persevere with the process. Striving for perfection can be extremely tough if you make it so. Your mind will tell you just how difficult it is if you allow it to. You must proceed without any negativity or you won't see results. Moving through the gears of life needs to be exciting and motivational, not weighed down by the kind of attitude that produces stress and anxiety. If you are loyal to the pillar of perseverance and develop a 'never give up' attitude, along with the other five pillars, incredible changes will occur in your life.

A reporter asked the inventor of the light bulb, Thomas Edison, 'How did it feel to fail 10,000 times?'

He replied, 'I didn't fail, I just found 10,000 ways that won't work!'

He also said, 'Many of life's failures are people who did not realise how close they were to success when they gave up.'

6. ACCOUNTABILITY

For me this is partnered with honesty. For a while, I toyed with the idea of replacing the word accountability with ownership. My thinking was, that in order to be honest with ourselves we must own and take responsibility for all that's going on within us. We have the ability to alter our pathway, including the way we think about things. That alone is a hugely challenging mission but to start with, we must own, or be accountable for, our inner 'current state of play' no matter what it is.

We avoid so many things in our lives rather than just owning them and dealing with them. Many of us are sensitive and defensive towards our actions and personal shortcomings and, at times, let ego stand in the way of truth. In some cases, to the point of a state of denial.

Holding yourself accountable at all times is actually both inspiring and liberating, and removing a blame ethos is transformational on its own. People who take responsibility for their actions, mistakes and failures know deep down that being accountable and owning them gives you the power to fix them. It's wonderful.

As Steve Maraboli, a behavioural scientist, says, *'For most people blaming others is a subconscious mechanism for avoiding accountability. In reality the only thing in your way is you.'*

I have also discovered that many people, particularly those who suffer with low self-esteem, find it difficult to own success and achievement and feel awkward receiving compliments and acknowledgements. Being accountable in life opens a gateway to a different world, allowing you to accept and acknowledge your own accomplishments. It also tends to erode the need to be judgemental of others.

Own your state of play, and tell the world what you have committed yourself to. When you add, honesty, trust, commitment, discipline and perseverance to accountability, you will be able to achieve any goal you set.

So, going back to the karate student who is always being adjusted and pushed forwards to achieve better stances, hands and feet positions and more *kime*. (*Kime* is a Japanese martial arts term meaning both power and focus. It is the ability to deliver maximum focussed energy on a target in a split second.) A growth mindset helps the student to deal with constant correction and to adopt the right attitude towards progression. Only 2% make it to black belt and 50% of karate students drop out at the white belt stage. If it was easy, we would all be living a black belt life! It's not easy, believe me, but anything can be achieved with the right mindset.

So those are the six pillars of the way. It is said that there are no guarantees in life, but success is guaranteed if you adhere to them.

You can employ the six pillars to many applications for setting goals. Let me tell you how one of my clients used them as a tool to reach his own goal. I began coaching him through some personal challenges and we re-engineered his belief structure into a platform ready to accept life-changing goals.

This client has operated in the world of high-end luxury for the last twenty-five years. After a while it became clear that his ambition to become a Chief Operating Officer (COO) for a global brand produced the right motivation.

He was asked to attend a high-level interview for the dream position of COO with the board of directors in Geneva, Switzerland. We had a session together prior to him travelling.

'How do I structure my pitch to them,' he asked.

I replied, 'Why not use the six pillars?'

The organisation was experiencing a number of operational challenges so we came up with this pitch. Here are the bullets.

- **HONESTY** – it's clear to everyone that the company is experiencing problems, therefore it is critical that we all be brutally honest with each other to obtain the much-needed clarity.
- **TRUST** – for our dreams to come to fruition we must trust each other totally.
- **COMMITMENT** – we have put together a challenging business plan (he walked everyone through it) and we will not achieve anywhere close to it unless each one of us commits 100%. We have to be 'all in'.
- **DISCIPLINE** – we must design new processes, a new way to operate with a clear structure and strategic objectives, revisit our core values and create the culture of togetherness and success. We will never see results if we are all doing our own thing based on our own values and beliefs. Therefore, it is critical we are disciplined and stick with a new way of doing things.
- **PERSEVERANCE** – it's going to be tough going but we must never give up, never throw the towel in. We must persevere.
- **ACCOUNTABILITY** – each and every one of us must own their role within this team and own it with pride. We are all accountable to our positions, each other and the organisation and with that level of attitude and commitment we will achieve our goals.

It was a magnificent pitch.

Not long after I received a text saying I'm COO.

A word of encouragement, guys…

Neuroscience (the study of the nervous system, focussing on the brain and its impact on behaviour) provides us with a weapon to support the transformation process, and we will unpack this in more detail later on in your journey. Our brains age with us but do not wither away to the extent many thought up until a few decades ago. We can truly generate new ways of thinking and behaving, new habits, and a new outlook to create change no matter how old we are. We can achieve almost anything we put our minds to.

So, there you have it. Before we go to your first grading to achieve white belt status, I want to recommend an audiobook I have listened to many times; *The Four Agreements* by Don Miguel Ruiz. It is based on ancient Toltec wisdom and covers the source of self-limiting beliefs. The Toltec were a tribe of people that lived in central Mexico before the Aztecs, from the 8th to the 12th century AD. One of the meanings of Toltec is 'cultured person'. *The Four Agreements* is a code of conduct that fits perfectly with living a black belt life.

I'll let you listen to it, or read it, and make your own judgements. For me, it offered some solutions to my personal inner battles. Being driven and competitive, I want to achieve something every day, but as with all of us, sometimes for no reason we just can't perform at our best.

In the book, the fourth agreement is 'always do your best'. My interpretation is that sometimes we wake up on five or six out of ten on our personal performance scale. As opposed to pushing ourselves until we break, or feeling that we have underachieved, the fourth agreement offers an alternative; it's OK, as long as I have done my best. Some days we are a Ferrari and some days a family saloon, we can reach our desired destination in both.

On the day of a karate grading the officiating sensei takes all the students for pre-grading training which covers their particular syllabus. So, to help you prepare and warm-up for your gradings I will recap the main points covered in the syllabus at the end of each chapter. Here is the first.

WHITE BELT GRADING WARM-UP:

The purpose of this syllabus was to introduce you to a process that I have named 'the way' taken from the translation of the word 'dojo' – 'the place of the way'. It was also to point out that all of us have vast reserves of untapped potential locked away in the cellars of our souls. It's there, guaranteed, but we must focus on some fundamental requirements to prepare for the inner adventure you're about to experience on the way to living a black belt life. Everything starts with our thinking, our choice of thought and how our attitude determines the response to various situations life pitches our way. This syllabus explains the need to appreciate that, just as in martial arts, it is critical to get the basics right first.

You will need to express yourself like never before and the results will be determined by how far you step outside of your comfort zone, stretching yourself and adopting a growth mindset with the aim of developing and growing as a human being. Therefore, the conclusion to the syllabus reverts to the beginning; 'attitude is everything'.

We looked at the significance of preparation, and a beautiful way to start and finish an experience using the tradition of *Mokuso*, a type of meditation to empty or clear the mind beforehand, touching on the wisdom of mindfulness and using reflection as another type of meditation to replay what's occurred.

And then there were the codes of respect as to how you should address and treat this book and your journey within it to maximise the benefits you will enjoy along the way.

We touched on Toltec wisdom and the book *The Four Agreements* by Don Miguel Ruiz. We examined Gichin Funakoshi's amazing twenty precepts and looked at creating new habits that, through hard work and repetition, will change our lives.

And, finally, you were introduced to the pivotal six pillars that will look after you throughout the adventure. Be loyal to them and everything will work out well.

Good luck with your grading. There are seven parts to it. Seven is an important number in Buddhism. Japanese Buddhists celebrate a baby's seventh day and mourn the seventh day after a person dies when the soul is said to cross over. In Japanese folklore there are the Shichifukujin, the Seven Gods of Luck.

WHITE BELT GRADING

1. Acquire a journal. This will become your 'book of life' for the rest of your life.
2. Read 'The Man in the Glass' again and note any resulting emotions.
3. Write down your interpretation of what 'spirit first – technique second' means to you.
4. Choose another two of the twenty precepts and bring together your own interpretation of them and how you can apply them to your life.
5. Attempt to bring *Mokuso* into your life. Try it for thirty seconds to start with, then build from there and note your feelings. Remember *Mokuso* is exercised in preparation for an event and as a tool of reflection after the event.
6. Revisit and learn the six pillars of the way as they will become your keys to transformation.
7. Write down your two main highlights/lessons/takeaways from the white belt syllabus.

Congratulations!
You are now a white belt.
Well done!

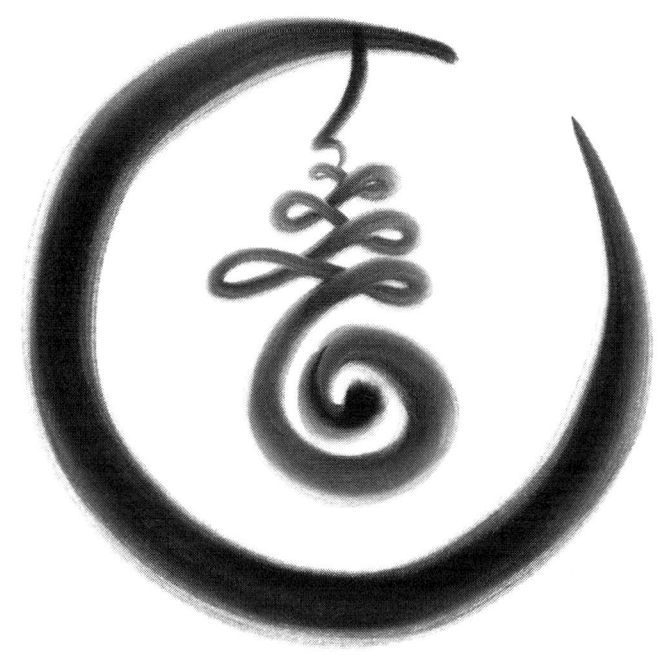

CHAPTER 2
ORANGE BELT
Cognitive Core Strength

'You have the power over your mind. Not outside events. Realise this and you will find strength.' ~ MARCUS AURELIUS

The Four Quadrants of Life

Physical
Mental
Emotional
Spiritual

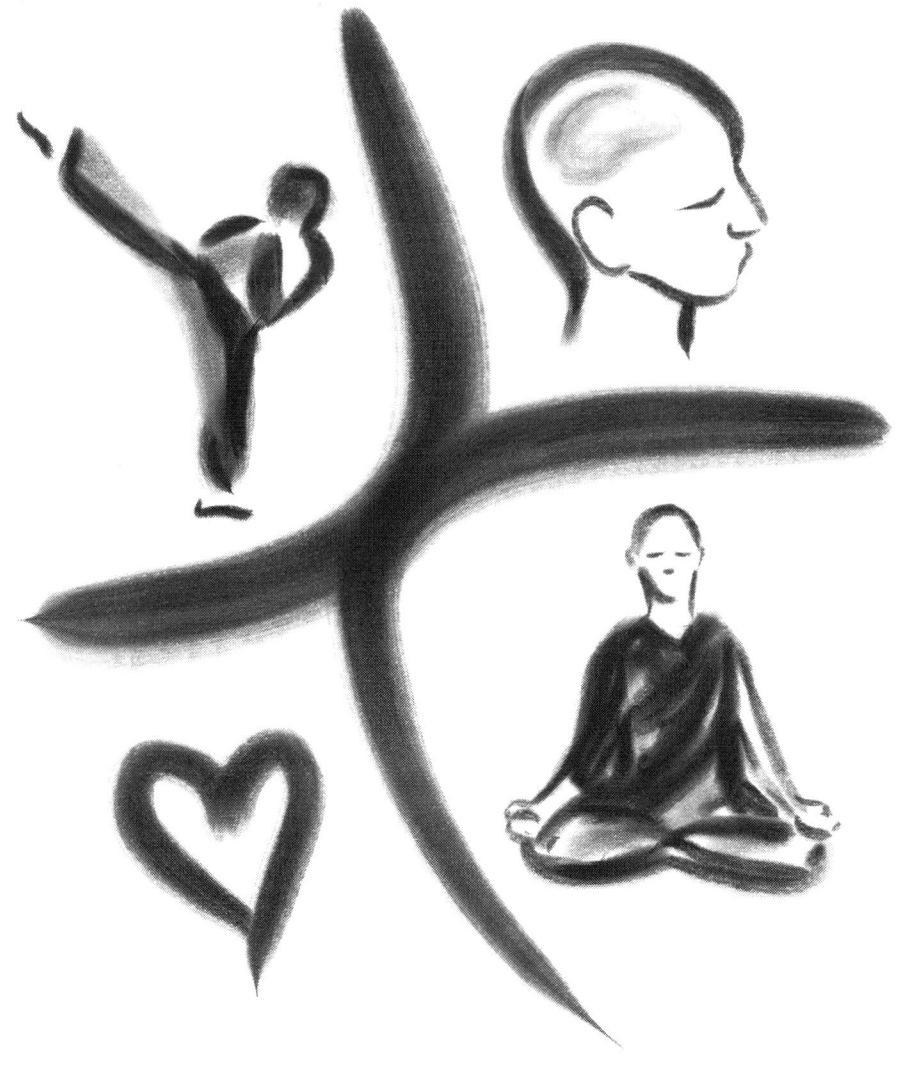

It can be argued that this is a very simplistic way to interpret our existence. The four quadrants are sometimes referred to as body, mind, soul and spirit.

However, when combined, these four elements form our attitude, actions and achievements. They enrich who we are and once we reach a better understanding and acceptance of them all, together with greater alignment and self-connection, both our inner and outer worlds become a better place to live. The resulting self-awareness and stronger life balance is when extraordinary things can be achieved. Each quadrant influences the other and, together, they become much greater than the sum of the parts. When in balance, they are integral to living a black belt life.

1. **PHYSICAL. The body. This is the part you can see. Physical wellness comes from physical health, fitness and care.**
2. **MENTAL. The human mind. A language that's made up of thoughts and imagination positive or negative. Our thinking moulds us into who we are.**
3. **EMOTIONAL. Emotions are made up from feelings triggered by thoughts and behaviour, stored memories and experiences. These can be positive or negative. Becoming in tune and aware of them helps control and regulation.**
4. **SPIRITUAL. This is built from faith, a divine belief and trust, but also self-belief and backing yourself, your instinct and finding your life purpose.**

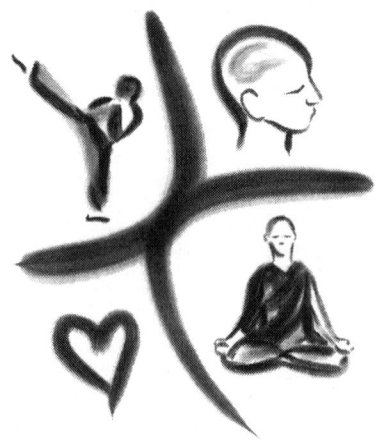

In the jigsaw puzzle of life, there are many little pieces that make that wonderful picture. No matter which way you look at it there will always be four parts which hold many pieces within.

In the world of martial arts, physical core strength is top of the agenda, and in plenty of other sports, too. It comes from targeting and strengthening the muscles in the torso to enable stability, posture, balance and stamina – the foundations required to perform well, ahead of so many other skills. Therefore, a great deal of effort and energy is applied to working on the physical aspects of core strength. Mastering these basics means progress can be made more quickly, safely and effectively, reducing your chances of injury.

But what about mental, emotional and spiritual core strength? Surely these are equally important? Actually, they are significantly more important. Mental strength, attitude and self-belief are what makes a winner and are the attributes that will enable you to become a black belt.

So, for the orange belt syllabus we are going to focus on the hidden three of the four aspects of your body; mental, spiritual and emotional core strength. Although not visible, they are all massively powerful, feeding your personal belief system and forming a solid structure that creates a platform to build your life upon.

In truth, the three are all interlinked. Mental strength and a feel-good mindset will translate into greater emotional stability, just as a pumped-out chest, good posture and a positive outlook will provide a flow of energy that you have rarely experienced before. We hear it said that the mind is a muscle, a mental muscle that can, if you develop it, help you to see things differently and transport you to the place where dreams become reality. Think of it this way, the late, great Wayne Dyer, the self-help author and motivational speaker said, *'If you change the way you look at things, the things you look at change.'* Please take time to examine those words. We have the power to create change by choice and this book is saying to you don't wait until you lose something to create that change. Don't wait until something traumatic occurs to bring about change.

Self-esteem, self-confidence and self-belief make up our belief structure and, regrettably, millions of us suffer negatively with these aspects of our lives. There is a relationship between self-esteem and self-confidence. Self-esteem is measured by how much you like and value yourself, whereas it's said that competence equals confidence. However, this is not just about being confident in a particular skillset but being a confident person and we all know how challenging that becomes as we deal with, and react to, what life throws at us. It's difficult to understand when an elite sportsman, earning millions of pounds a year, is said to be suffering from a lack of confidence. We hear this all the time and it just highlights the fact that it can happen to anyone. It all starts and finishes with the mind. Our thinking. It's absolutely incredible. If there was just one thing I could achieve with this book, in terms of helping others, it would be to help grow and maintain their confidence, always aware they can scoop up more when it needs a top-up! To be confident means so much, I know. It's the greatest gift of all and a priceless asset.

When I reflect on that, growing people's confidence is what I do for a living. Although each of us has a brain, our minds are all different. We react differently to different things and we must be mindful that it's about how the person feels and not the event that's causing it. I want to share my own experiences with you as examples.

I had a good upbringing, working class and modest but I was afforded lots of love, affection and attention. When I look back, I was genuinely a happy child. However, I was small for my age and growing up I became very conscious of this. I was lucky that I was a good footballer as that kept the school bullies away from me as they respected my skills. That said, as soon as I took off my football kit and became a regular school student my lack of confidence surfaced again. I was told early on in my school years that music and, in particular, singing wasn't my forte. And if you stand by me at a wedding or a funeral today you will never hear me sing. I lip-sync to the hymns and songs. The message from that music teacher has remained in my subconscious all of my life.

Another example of how an event from the past can affect us for many years to come. My mum took me to the dentist regularly. If there was a problem with a tooth the dentist would paint it black. Yes, black. There must have been some science behind it. So, when I was around six or seven years old, she painted my top left incisor black. That was a shocker and it stopped me smiling. I was a super happy little boy, who suddenly stopped smiling. Some of you are exactly right when you think there's a lot worse that can happen in life than a black tooth and I'm the first to agree. But how did that one thing affect my confidence? I stopped smiling and laughing overnight and it went on for months and months. I felt ugly with a black tooth and when the school photographer appeared once a term I suffered with massive anxiety. It was horrible and all going on in my head. I only recently told my mum and I wish I hadn't, as it made her feel sad. And that black tooth left me with a crooked smile for the rest of my life.

A competent person is a confident person who can transition into a person with presence. But what does this mean? Presence could be described as an energy someone emits just by being there. We have all met people with presence. I have met a few in my time, for sure. My sensei described a moment when the great sensei – Keinosuke Enoeda, entered a restaurant he was in, and the hairs on the back of his neck stood up! Now I view that as having presence!

When your self-esteem is high it tends to positively affect the quality of your performance. When you perform well and achieve good results this in turn increases your self-esteem. So, the whole process becomes an upward spiral. It's amazing how this works.

Check in with yourself on a regular basis, to ascertain how well your confidence and self-esteem levels are performing. If they need a boost, then the tools we're about to discover will help you to reset and recharge them.

Throughout this book we will not veer from the inside-out approach to self-development, with the aim of creating the best version of yourself. To discover exactly what you have in your tank in the form of potential and how we can access what you have stored away.

As you move through the grades, you will start to understand and appreciate more, the power of the mind and how you can use this to influence your feelings and behaviour. This idea is backed up by neuroscience. Certain situations produce neurotransmitters, sometimes referred to as chemical messages, triggered by the brain in various situations which effect psychological functions such as fear, joy, pleasure and our moods. This process will help you to understand the natural routes to this group of neurochemicals that can alter and influence your mindset and behaviour. I read an article published by the charity 'A Lust for Life' that referred to these neurochemicals as a D.O.S.E. of happiness, a great way to describe them.

Here is D.O.S.E.

D – DOPAMINE

Referred to as the happy hormone, dopamine is a neurotransmitter that plays a role in how happy we feel. It is released by the brain when we are expecting or receiving a reward which produces a surge of pleasure. It can cause excitement and energy when triggered. Dopamine is a key aspect in the goal-setting process covered later. A word of caution, a dopamine hit doesn't last long and leaves us desiring more. This can lead to bad habits due to its addictive nature.

O – OXYTOCIN

The love hormone that is secreted by the brain in romantic engagements and, like dopamine, it sends signals throughout the entire body to reward certain behaviours. It also plays a part in bonding such as childbirth and social connection. A hug can produce oxytocin hence its nickname 'cuddle hormone'. Unlike dopamine oxytocin will produce a feeling of calmness and safety.

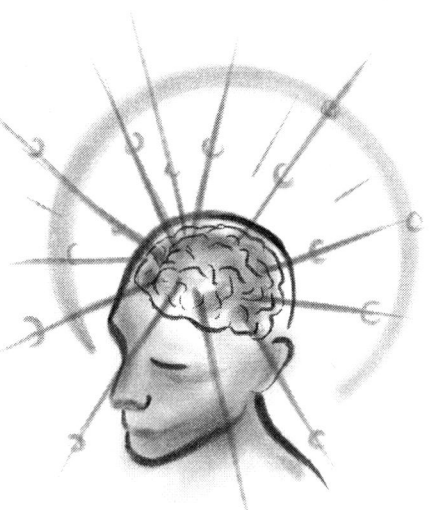

S – SEROTONIN

As a neurotransmitter, serotonin helps to regulate happiness and moods and plays a big part in our confidence and belief structure. Due to the power of the mind, we can raise our levels of serotonin without physically doing anything. It plays a vital role in self-acceptance. We will return to this again in a higher grade in the book. Serotonin also plays a part in our digestion and sleep patterns. When we feel respected and important we receive a hit of serotonin.

E – ENDORPHINS

Our innate painkiller. Endorphins, when released, increase our feelings of well-being and pleasure. It is a special neurotransmitter that provides a double hit of reduction in pain and increase in pleasure. Endorphins can be released through exercise. A great workout can produce a feeling of euphoria hence the expression 'runners' high'.

Let's now start to develop a bulletproof belief structure that will guarantee delivery of those feel-good hormones. The definition of a belief system or structure is 'a set of principles that together form the basis of a moral code'. This, for me, is an incredibly accurate definition. A great deal has been written about belief systems, but I want to share with you my personal approach, which I have seen, first-hand, deliver astonishing results.

Building Your Fortress

Before anything can be achieved, you must cultivate a mental, emotional and spiritual strength that will be the foundation on which to build a more confident and triumphant future. This process is made up of seven parts and I have called this the fortress model. A fortress is a strong building or group of buildings that can be defended from attack. With this analogy I use the fortress as a defence against attack from our negative thinking and emotions when responding to certain events in our lives. The model is made up of seven fundamental structures, all immensely important but they become much stronger and more powerful when aligned together. They form a secure defence system not susceptible to outside influence or disturbance.

The lucky number seven again features as it brings with it something extra special. The seven parts that make up the fortress model combine to deliver an immensely powerful inner strength, a faith and mindset, that triggers a shift in self-esteem, confidence and belief.

This is the first stage of the inside-out living philosophy of this book that will help you transition to a better or new version of yourself. It's in your hands now!

THE FORTRESS MODEL

1. Core values
2. Gratitude
3. Life achievements
4. Self-kindness
5. Giving back
6. Self-limitations
7. Facing fears

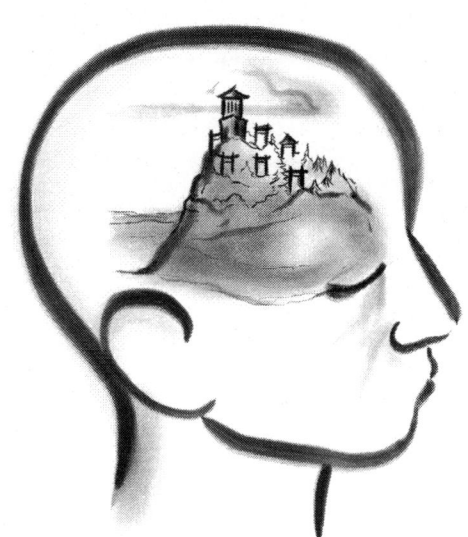

1. CORE VALUES

A core value is a fundamental belief or practice as to how you conduct your life. It can be applied to an individual, team or organisation.

Our core values represent who we strive to be and our own beliefs. Together they form a private navigation system that takes us to the life destinations of our choosing and beyond. They are an inner GPS or compass, an instinctive guidance and defence system.

Firstly, we have to revisit or rediscover our values and remind ourselves of what they are. We have to take them out of storage and give them a good mental polish. Some people have archived their values, others are not even aware they have them or have ever considered them to be the framework of a belief structure.

Uncovering your core values is the first of the seven parts to this system. They will look slightly different for everyone. Having decided what they are, you will then need to put them in order of significance. Give it some thought – what is your ultimate guiding principle?

Each and every client I have coached has completed this exercise. The most wonderful thing is that when their value system is unpacked, there is always one value standing out and staring back that will steer them through a particular challenge. Together your values make up a type of raw wisdom that becomes your trusted advisor. There will be a value that always finds the way forward.

One client, who was a business owner, worked hard on himself over a period of time. In our second meeting we extracted his values. Initially they were:

1. Passion
2. Commitment
3. Helpfulness
4. Generosity
5. Curiosity
6. Practicality
7. Fairness

During our journey, we discovered there were parts missing in his leadership skills that he felt were adversely impacting on the business. We later found the parts were directness, confidence and assertiveness. We agreed to drop these values into his system with the condition that he was loyal to them and he consciously lived by his values every day. Over time, his leadership style started to change, as did his outlook. It goes without saying that the business started to show improved performance levels.

Once we are aware of our value systems and appreciate them, they become one of the first tools of life. As mentioned earlier, they become our compass. You can strengthen your value structure when you discover more about yourself. You can, as the business owner did, add to your list with the proviso that you are totally committed to your additions. It won't work if you're not.

I worked with another client who suffered horrendously with low self-confidence and self-esteem. Believe me when I say they were at rock bottom. When we first met she marked them both 2/10. When we unpacked her values she put 'hardworking' at number one. She described herself as 'a grafter'. Accountability was another one in her top five. During our first meeting I pointed towards her number one value and said that if she applied it to our journey together then her life will change. I witnessed an immediate change to her persona. It created a mini-epiphany and gave her the much-needed clarity she already possessed – the tool to help her change. She committed to work hard to change her life.

My number one value is passion. It's said passion is the fuel of life, the fuel that keeps the fire for life burning. This is one of my favourite quotes of all-time and I live by this.

'There is no passion to be found playing small – in settling for a life that is less than you are capable of.' ~ NELSON MANDELA

2. GRATITUDE

It is said that feeling gratitude, described as a positive emotional response, has healing powers. Gratitude is observing and acknowledging goodness in the world. It reduces pain, improves well-being and allows you to be more present in the moment. It has also been described as a natural antidepressant. It produces positive emotions and optimism. Gratitude alone is so powerful; it can change everything. Many people start and finish their days by stating or recording in their journal a number of things they are grateful for.

There is a beautiful video called 'A Good Day' by Brother David Steindl-Rast, a Benedictine monk. He dives deep into how gratitude can be perceived. Gratitude helps us to find reflection and balance in our lives. He says, *'If you're grateful you're not in fear.'*

It's easy to say we should be grateful, or that we are grateful, but do we really feel it deep inside of us? Do we experience the gift and presence of gratitude within us? When we do, it reveals itself with an inner warmth, a glow of thankfulness and ultimately being grateful makes us happy. The benefits are endless! Research has shown that it reduces stress, including depression, improves general well-being and strengthens relationships. The more grateful we are, the happier we become. It's a fact and there is scientific evidence to support this.

Showing or expressing gratitude releases two of the aforementioned neurotransmitters; dopamine and serotonin. They enhance our mood, make us feel happy and contribute to the warm feelings of closeness and positive connections. Gratitude destroys negative thinking but has to be practised and perfected.

'Acknowledging the good that you already have in your life is the foundation for all abundance.' ~ ECKHART TOLLE

3. LIFE ACHIEVEMENTS

Revisiting all the successes in our lives, from the smallest to the most earth shattering, is so powerful for our confidence and self-esteem. Over time, we forget what it feels like to be successful. Whether it's passing your driving test, running a marathon, giving birth to your first child, fighting an illness or achieving a promotion at work. Whatever it is, however it could be framed, it's still an achievement, and we all need to shout from the rooftops about our successes.

One of my clients had to work really hard to find any successes to speak of, but once he started, they just flowed. I watched him describe winning an international work-related award which, incredibly, he'd forgotten about. As he was describing the event to me, he recalled his name being called out as the winner of the award and I noticed him rubbing his arms. I asked what he was doing, and he said he had goosebumps. That exercise alone produced such a positive and emotional response. This was from a person who was suffering with clinical depression and had been prescribed huge doses of antidepressants.

When was the last time you checked into your success résumé? I bet it's been years since you reviewed it. When you revisit these events in your mind you can create similar emotional responses through reactive neurochemistry. This will be covered in more detail later on, along with how past reflection and future visualisation can be transformed into further tools for your kitbag of life. To appreciate how this works, you need to understand that the brain is a prediction machine which assumes everything that has happened in our past will reoccur in the future. It has to work so much harder to create something from nothing so uses past experiences to calculate from. So, if you focus on the detail of past successes and apply what you have learnt from the failures, it bodes well for a successful future.

'The roots of true achievement lie in the will to become the best that you can become.' ~ HAROLD TAYLOR

4. SELF-KINDNESS

In the first three of the seven points, I'm nudging you outside your personal safe zone. With this element I'm not nudging you, I'm dragging you! I know from many years of coaching that no one likes this next exercise; no one enjoys revealing the things they like about themselves. However, once they get out of their own way, people start to embrace it. Then they're off, and I can't stop them.

It's time to shine the torch of life back towards you and start to focus on much-needed me-time. Why do we give ourselves such a hard time? Some of us are extremely vocal about it too, talking about our flaws, our weaknesses and our idiosyncrasies, but never our strengths, our skills or our quirks. Our positive attributes. To reinforce our belief structure, this fourth part needs to be as solid as the rest.

This exercise, finding out things you like about yourself, is a liberating and fulfilling experience, but every exercise needs practice if you're to become a master at it. This part of the fortress model helps you feel good about yourself from the inside out as well as the outside in. Happiness is not found in the outer world – it's positioned right next to self-esteem, confidence, motivation and mindfulness – they're all inside jobs.

I've asked everyone I've ever worked with to complete this exercise. I watch them writhing with embarrassment as I set this for their homework as part of the coaching process. When they arrive for their next session with their list in their hand, they're already in a different mindset. Everyone starts with a modest tone, but after a few examples I have the pleasure of watching my clients start to uncover all the things they like and admire about themselves. In the past they have been afraid or too humble to ever mention these incredible qualities and characteristics. Many clients even mentioned that they couldn't help but smile during this process, which was incredible as some were struggling with deep-rooted self-confidence issues.

On your journey to black belt living, it's essential to revisit your list and see if other things can be added; things you have learnt about yourself that you didn't know before.

'You are very powerful, provided you know how powerful you are.'
~ YOGI BHAJAN

5. GIVING BACK

What do you give back? How can you give back?

All of us need to give something back to life, help someone or a cause. It's so important for all the obvious reasons but also for our own personal well-being. Doing things for others helps boost our mood, reduces stress and benefits our mental health. Again, this has been scientifically proven to benefit the giver more than the receiver in terms of creating personal joy and a feel-good factor.

Helping others diverts attention away from ourselves, producing those wonderful neurotransmitters of dopamine, serotonin and oxytocin that create the feeling of happiness! It's a clear win-win scenario, so shouldn't we be doing it more?

Even opening a door for someone or letting someone in front of you in a queue will produce that feel-good factor. Just one simple act of kindness can reduce stress and is scientifically proven to reduce blood pressure! Add to that a boost in self-esteem and you could begin to reverse some of the challenges of mental health.

In karate there is a culture of helping others. I often see higher grades helping lower grades, always volunteering to help teach, train and give advice and tips. You see black belts helping white belts with the same laser-focussed attention they apply when instructing a class or being trained themselves. Black belts recognise this attitude is a part of their code of continual growth. I just love this philosophy; it is quite unique in my experience.

A white belt looks to their right and sees the line of coloured belts as a journey of greatness to the place where the black belts stand. So, looking right is the way ahead, whereas the black belt looks to the left and sees the journey they have been on. This is what creates this unparalleled environment of help and support. No matter how good you are, whatever your status, everyone started as a white belt. This is a deep-rooted and fundamental ethic within the dojo, the place of the way.

'Non nobis solum nati sumus.' ~ MARCOS TULLIUS CICERO (NOT FOR OURSELVES ALONE ARE WE BORN).

6. SELF-LIMITATIONS

Firstly, we need to identify our limitations and be honest about them. It's using the first success pillar from the white belt syllabus, honesty, and again this is a liberating exercise.

Are our limitations real or potential limitations, and are they getting in the way of achieving what we are capable of?

There is a formula used in some coaching arenas: p=P-I. It stands for 'performance equals potential minus interference' (p=P-I). It raises the question as to what is actually interfering and stopping us from being able to access our potential.

Most people perform below their potential, doing less than they are capable of, and this simple formula helps us find the answer.

So, what gets in the way? We do!

The biggest obstacles are placed in front of us by ourselves. Negative thinking, self-judgement, loss of discipline or focus, fears, doubts and procrastination. This leads to low confidence and poor self-esteem, as we covered earlier. This is not an arena for high performance.

So, how do we get out of the way? Well, doing exactly this exercise – starting with an honest self-appraisal. Once you have completed this you will already have begun the process. Once you are aware of something, particularly if you write it down, the dynamic changes and you are on your way.

Ask yourself the following questions. What are your limitations? What is standing in your way? What does elite performance look like?

7. FACING FEARS

We need to experience fear. It's our survival mechanism and is covered in more detail in the yellow belt syllabus. Basically, we feel fear as the brain's number one priority is to keep us alive – at all times.

Facing your fears and understanding them provides you with another layer of armour in your belief structure. As I said, we need our survival system fully functioning as a response to threat and danger from the outside world. But it's the threat and danger from the inner world that's the real issue, but this is something we can learn to recognise, manage and, ultimately, change.

To start with, we must realise that many of our fears are not actually dangerous, for example, public speaking. It's said people fear public speaking more than death! Fear of failure, fear of rejection and fear of the unknown when stepping out of your comfort zone aren't necessarily dangerous – just a bit scary.

Fear is another form of self-limitation that inhibits you and holds you back. It can even stop your progress altogether. Facing your fears will instinctively help you to cope with them better and eventually overcome them. However, avoiding them will only increase and compound anxiety. The brain has to experience repeated exposure to fear in order to overcome it.

When I coach people, we look to change the language of our dialogue relating to fear. For example, replacing the word 'fear' with 'challenge'. It makes it easier to talk about. Then we evaluate the challenge in a sort of a risk versus reward assessment. Of course, there are levels of fear that transcend into phobia which has a far greater strength and energy.

In facing your fears, you have taken the first step. You might well find that the other six parts of the fortress model will help you to deal with, and overcome, them.

There it is, there is the model to design and build your belief structure, your own belief fortress. It's yours and yours alone and will protect you against both your outer enemies and, our greatest challenge, our inner enemies. The mind trash so many of us experience on a daily basis.

Now, please note this, as it is vitally important. The fortress model, just like any fortress, can be enhanced and strengthened over time. New structures can be added to toughen its walls of protection but also make it more comfortable to live within. You can add more to your value system when you discover new things about yourself. These should be dropped in as, remember, these are a reflection of who you really are. Then your achievements will extend, as will your gratitude, you'll find more things you like about yourself, and, of course, what you give back to life will also change. As these aspects of your life expand and develop your fears and limitations will diminish.

The author Diana Gaboldon said:

'...it's as though everyone has a small place inside themselves, maybe, a private bit they keep to themselves. It's like a little fortress, where the most private part of you lives – maybe it's your soul, maybe just that bit makes you yourself and not anyone else.'

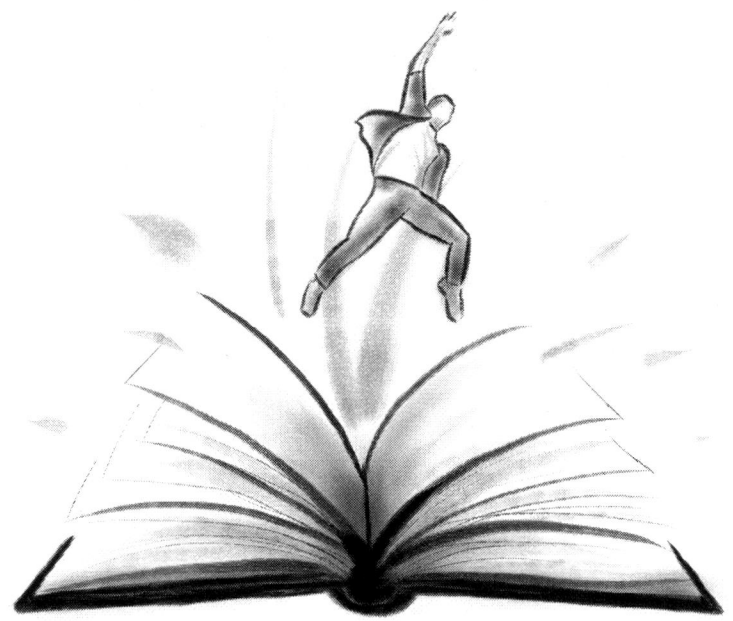

How well does that capture my fortress model?

I encourage all my clients to invest in a beautiful journal to keep a log of their coaching journey. In it I ask them to record the learning gained, any new tools and rituals, not forgetting those brightly polished life-changing goals, as well as the insightful 'aha' moments. This was the first task in your white belt grading. It's so important to buy into the journaling concept and equally important to jot down in it your own fortress model, point by point. As I have just mentioned, keep building on it, and adding to it. It's so incredibly powerful. I call this type of journaling building a 'book of life', as the notes always truthfully reflect who you are and are an accurate measurement of progress.

In my own journal, I have also included some of my favourite quotes, mantras and affirmations as well as my belief structure, my personal fortress. I can see my limitations every time I open it so I can face them, be honest about them, then develop them into strengths. I have penned a couple of personal supportive notes to myself, and written down how I can give something back to others, how I can be of help. I have also included the following statement: 'Before the sun sets, do one more thing that helps you get closer to your goal'.

Over time, I have developed my 'book of life' to become a fundamental part of my life and my coaching system. The 'book of life' really does develop into an authentic reflection of you. No one else but you. It represents who you are, your strengths, values, successes, goals and special personal notes that contribute to your self-growth as a human being.

I recommend to my clients that they check in with their book regularly. I used to say to them, 'Whenever there's a challenge in your life, open the book and check your value system as there will be one staring at you to help you overcome the particular obstacle you are facing.' Now, it's evolved into, 'When something nice or abundant happens check in with your book, look at your values and there will be one staring at you that will illustrate why this happened.' That's why I call it the 'book of life'. It really does help you deal with the pushes and pulls we all face. The brilliant Jim Rohn said:

'The same wind blows on us all, the winds of disaster, opportunity and change. Therefore, it is not the blowing of the wind but the setting of the sails that will determine our direction in life.'

My 'book of life' is my rudder, navigation and protection system. Your book can help you take control of the journey, and even change the course, to enable you to reach your goal. It's a magnificent personal tool. Totally unique as there's only one of you and, therefore, it's the only one in existence. A quote by the author Irene C Kassorla sums it up, *'The pen that writes your life story must be held in your own hand.'*

Remember it's not a diary – it's your DNA. DNA stands for Deoxyribonucleic acid and is defined as a molecule that contains the instructions an organism needs to develop. Your book is the molecule, and it too should become a living thing, always evolving with additions to strengthen the belief system and notable achievements, events and things that are positively influencing your life. The 'book of life' doesn't only have to be there for you when things go wrong, it's simply your go-to whenever you feel like checking-in.

I can't tell you how important it is to building that belief system. It will stay with you for the rest of your life, it will follow you wherever you go and will be the foundation for discovering many other wonders within a new world of excitement, growth and abundance.

The magnificent Wayne Dyer, self-help and spiritual author, tells this story:

There was a wise, old cat and a small kitten in an alleyway. The old cat saw the kitten chasing its tail and asked, 'Why are you chasing your tail?'

The kitten replied, 'I've been attending cat philosophy school and I have learnt that the most important thing for a cat is happiness, and that happiness is located in my tail. Therefore, I am chasing it: and when I catch it, I shall have happiness forever.'

Laughing, the wise, old cat replied, 'My son, I wasn't lucky enough to go to cat philosophy school, but as I've gone through life, I too have realised that the most important thing for a cat is happiness, and indeed that it is located in my tail. The difference I've found though, is that whenever I chase after it, it keeps running away from me, but when I go about my business and live my life, it just seems to follow after me wherever I go.'

I love the wisdom in that story and, like everything in this book, it's about continuous growth through self-reflection and self-development. Like the story of the cat's tail, let your 'book of life' follow you wherever you go. No matter who you are we can all keep learning and growing as human beings. We should be grateful for this alone.

ORANGE BELT GRADING WARM-UP:

So, to recap where we are as we arrive at the orange belt grading. The syllabus beautifully segues from what we learned in the white belt to building a rock-solid belief structure covering three of the four quadrants of life.

The mental aspect highlighted the need to bring more gratitude into our lives as well as starting to become kinder and more compassionate towards ourselves, introducing more of a positive note to our self-talk, while also facing our fears and limitations.

The emotional quadrant looked at various neurochemistry that's generated by certain situations and behaviour. Having a degree of understanding as to what's occurring and why automatically helps the control and regulation of emotions.

The spiritual side of the belief system framework embraced the notion of giving back, thinking of others and what we can do to help them. As a white belt we touched on meditation in terms of emptying our cup and tuning in to be more present. This is also a part of the spiritual element of the journey.

With these incredible life foundations in place, we can then design and build a way of living using the incredible tools that you will discover as you travel through the grades. This syllabus deliberately locates and stirs up some of those lost memories of achievement and takes us out of our zone of safety to dial in to our inner self. Probably for the first time in a long while, if not ever, it created some 'me-time'.

We homed into your value system bringing it back to life, lighting it up to become your spiritual beacon and personal GPS that will take you wherever you want to go.

Finally, we covered the lifelong benefits attached to creating your own 'book of life' and how yours will be the only one in existence.

Remember, it's important to check in with your emotions when completing the orange belt grading as you will be receiving D.O.S.E.s of neurochemistry along the way.

I wish you all the best.

ORANGE BELT GRADING

1.   Revisit 'The Man in the Glass' and write down any further insights it creates.
2.   List seven of your core values.
3.   Circle your number one core value then list them all in order of significance.
4.   Name the seven things you are most grateful for in your life.
5.   Write down seven of your life achievements. Again note and journal your emotions doing this exercise.
6.   Name seven things you like about yourself.
7.   Note your main self-limitations.
8.   What are the fears you currently live with?
9.   Name three occasions when you have helped someone recently. Note and journal the emotions generated doing this exercise.
10. Add a value that doesn't exist in your current value system, but you would like to add and be loyal to. This will make a difference to your direction and speed of transformation.

Well done! Your belief structure, your spiritual fortress has been created. And now your inner GPS now goes live!

Congratulations!
You have your orange belt.

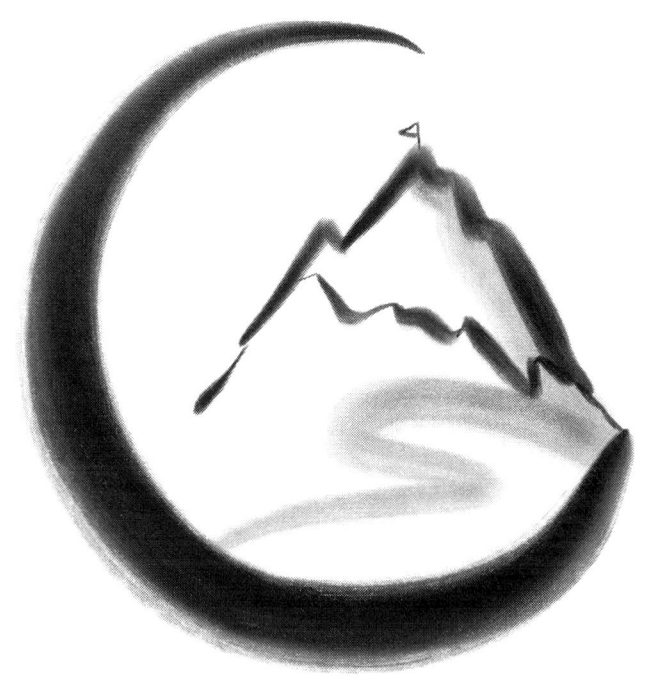

CHAPTER 3
RED BELT
The Secret to Goal Setting

'Dream, Believe, Dare, Do.' ~ WALT DISNEY

I'm going to start by asking you to make a mental note or write this down in your journal:

This belt is the most important of all – it's your launch pad!

This is the syllabus that will propel you to black belt and beyond. You are about to take a crucial step towards change. We have reached the critical stage of the journey, the part where I launch you into a new way of thinking and living. In fact, a way to design how you want your life to look. And you can do all of this by committing yourself to a goal-setting mindset. Whoever you are, wherever you are, if you get this part of the process right then your life will change instantaneously.

You should now have a robust belief system in place and this will get stronger over time, if you stick to the rules. Now I'm going to explain to you exactly how and why goal setting will guarantee success and separate you from the rest. You're about to join a new elite club and become one of the privileged few who can grasp and implement these life-changing skills.

OK here we go...

Let's start with a little neuroscience. The brain-organising principle is threat or reward; however, there are five times as many threat circuitries, so it doesn't take much for the brain to be sent into danger mode.

Test yourself, ask someone to give you honest feedback on something you did or said. Check your emotions and acknowledge the feelings you're experiencing. That uneasiness or awkwardness is because your brain has moved into threat mode. Understanding that the brain has a bias towards negativity and fear, explains why some of us are prevented from committing seriously to challenging goals, for fear of failure and fear of rejection. As humans, these are our greatest fears.

The flip side to this is that the brain loves certainty, so it loves a plan with clarity – clear, concise steps to its destination. We are hardwired to seek it. We spend our lives trying to predict the future, yet the truth is it's impossible. So, we have to do it manually.

Even though the brain is extremely complex and still has much untapped learning to be discovered it prefers to focus on a problem it has already met because it finds it easier to process events that have already taken place. The brain recognises a past incident as something real, rather than having to find a solution for something that's based in the future — and is therefore not yet real. The future has to be created through thought and this process takes up much more energy. Essentially, the brain is seeking efficiency — the easiest option.

Clarity is the key to many things and in goal setting it's absolutely vital! Uncertainty brings with it worry and anxiety. Again, do a little self-reflection and think about how you felt when you were faced with uncertainty in your life. It's really hard to deal with, isn't it?

I hate to say it, but that's why we all know people who moan a lot. These people are letting their brains run riot, focussing on what they perceive are problems and threats as opposed to working a little harder to find solutions, positivity and things that make them happy. It's so much easier to choose the lazy option.

Goal setting can be an effective brain hack that helps us cut through the negative bias that we are hardwired to default to, generating immediate positivity — yes, literally straight away. We will cover negative bias in more detail as we advance through the belts. Don't get me wrong, the goal-setting process needs initial heavy mental flexing but like a rocket launching into space, it uses most of its fuel to muscle through the gravitational pull and then lets momentum and guidance take it to its destination. Goal setting is a similar process. If you're prepared to put the effort in up front, the rewards can be beyond anything you thought possible.

In short, everything we do is based on our brain's drive to minimise the threat of danger and maximise reward. When certainty is met, we instantly feel better. In David Rock's book, *The Brain at Work,* he refers to smartphones as 'dopamine delivery devices' in that they provide certainty very quickly on various topics such as the weather, traffic or the latest news. Certainty at our fingertips and our brains like certainty!

Here's a little warning to keep in mind…there is a danger that, through our thinking, we can create self-delusion or a false reality. Therefore, your goals must manifest from deep, pure, honest belief. First and foremost, they have to be conceivable to be achievable. Only then can you begin to design invincible routes to accomplish them, and only then will you enjoy those amazing sensations of confidence and certainty, which it has been argued is actually the same thing.

So, if you apply yourself properly and stick to the process, incorporating the six pillars of the way detailed in this book and, in particular, number six – accountability, I promise you will reach places you have only dreamt about.

It's an interesting fact that human beings are the only life form on the planet with the capability to alter the course of their life. As humans we have the ability to change our life purpose, our journey and our ultimate destination all by setting defined goals. As my coach and great friend David TS Wood said, *'You can live life by design.'*

So, let's design your life.

Ask yourself these seven questions:

1. **What would you love to do, to change?**
2. **Where do you want to be?**
3. **What do you want to accomplish?**
4. **What is important to you?**
5. **What is your life mission?**
6. **How far do you believe you can go?**
7. **What do you dream about?**

Work out what success looks like to you. Get creative, get imaginative and start to design a new way of life. Now we are starting to look forward and not dwell on or live in the past and we're definitely not going to be stuck or stand still. The past is gone, there is only one way to go. It's said, 'if you stand still, you go backwards'. So, from this moment on, using the rocket metaphor, we have lift-off!

Why am I making such a big deal about goals? What do they really offer? What is so incredibly important about them? Can they truly help you to transform your life? Why am I talking and writing about them as if they were some sort of magical manifestation?

Well, I want to share with you what they offer and precisely how and why the process I'm about to reveal can cultivate wonderful things – deliver the fairy tale – but only if you're prepared to do the work! I will show you the way but you are the one that will have to walk it.

Goals are exciting and exhilarating, they enrich life in a way that's difficult to put into words, yet perfectly described in a quote by Benjamin Mays: 'The tragedy of life doesn't lie in not reaching your goal. The tragedy lies in having no goals to reach.'

What are the benefits of having goals? Honestly, there are too many to mention but you will receive an endless supply of life-changing paybacks. They give you clarity, certainty and control over what the future looks like, which you all now know the brain thrives on. They prevent us from getting set in our ways and simply wandering through life. They stretch, test and challenge us and provide a high level of meaning, purpose and motivation. If it's framed correctly, constructing a goal creates up an upward spiral of positivity. Once your goal is set and you start to think about it, the magic of neurochemistry kicks in. You will be buzzing from the get-go, which in turn makes you focus even more on your goal, which makes you feel even more positive and inspired and so on. On your journey to achieving your overall goal you will also receive many smaller hits of accomplishment; enjoyable little wins. These are like bursts of mental sunshine that we all need as we take on the pushes and pulls of life.

Goals should and must challenge your potential, taking you outside your safe zone into an exciting space of learning and development that results in fulfilment, pride and the opportunity to achieve higher levels of confidence and self-esteem. When you combine all these positives, it harvests happiness. Surely, this has got to be everyone's ultimate goal? Jane Fonda said, 'It's never too late to start over, never too late to be happy.' I couldn't agree more.

A goal could be set in the outer world as a material prize or focussed on the inner self such as personal growth. Either way, the effect of setting the process in motion to achieve either of them will be life-changing.

Some people translate goals into pressure, they flip them to a negative mindset, approaching them as if they're a weight or burden. Subsequently, they resist the much-needed effort and commitment to create new routines and habits. I have worked with clients who interpret goals like this but still constantly search for change in their lives. Einstein said, 'Insanity is people doing the same thing over and over and expecting different results.' Just think about that for a moment. Whereas Henry Ford said, 'If you always do what you've always done, you'll always get what you've always got.'

It is said 'you cannot hit a target if you cannot see it'. How true. That's why it is so important to have goals to aim for and the belief that you can hit them. You can also hit a moving target, by the way, if you focus on it enough, and that's a very important point in this syllabus.

The trouble is that many people leave goal setting until 31st December every year. 'I'm giving up smoking', 'I'm going to lose weight', 'I'm going to get fit', 'I'm changing my diet', 'I'm getting a new job', 'I'm going to earn more money' and so on. Every year millions of goals are set as New Year's resolutions and, guess what, around 80% fail in the first month. So, why is that? Why are we great at goal setting and rubbish at goal getting? Why can't we stick it out? Why can't we stand true to our commitment, why do we slip and constantly fail?

Lack of discipline, or 'willpower' if you'd like to call it that, is certainly a contributory factor but there are other fundamental flaws in the goal commitment and our attitude towards it that result in failure. When it comes to New Year's resolutions, many of them are goals to give up something; for example, giving up smoking, stropping drinking alcohol and quitting eating certain foods. This causes the brain to perceive this type of challenge as a threat. It's 'giving up' something, which is negative, not being 'given' something, which is a positive and therefore a reward. Now you can appreciate why the stereotypical New Year's resolutions fail most of the time

As I explained in the introduction, in 2001 I walked into the dojo for the first time. I stood at the far left-hand end of the room looking down the long line, through the various belt colours, to where the elite, the black belts, were standing. I honestly believe there is no better example of a planned and laid-out goal. The line provided visibility, clarity, a clear process, steps of accomplishment and a clear timeline also.

And now I'm going to explain how you can use this bulletproof process to achieve your goals without needing to enter a dojo.

WHAT IS A GOAL?

Wikipedia states, 'A goal is an idea of the future or desired result that a person or a group of people envision, plan and commit to achieve.'

In my own language and thinking paradigm the Wikipedia version is referring to an objective not a goal. This is my personal version of what a goal is: 'A goal is an inspirational challenge outside the zone of comfort that when accomplished impacts life in a truly positive way.'

Goals are not deleting 100 emails by 9.00 am, doing the shopping, walking the dog, being on time for meetings and getting through 'to do' lists. These are simply tasks. A goal is something that has an outcome that can alter your life. It inspires you to the point that when you think about it you get goosebumps. It's exhilarating not tiresome, it's inspiring not boring, it's positive not a pressure.

Remember, this is my definition of a goal. This book is all about your interpretation and what works best for you. You will convert much of the content of this book in your own private and unique way in order to become the best version of yourself. That's just perfect! That's exactly what I'm hoping for.

Coach David TS Wood said to me once, 'When you get goosebumps about something you know it's right.' I've never forgotten that, and I use it all the time when coaching clients, in particular when a client has a breakthrough or epiphany.

When I looked down that line of coloured belts in the dojo, it was crystal clear what I had to do to reach my destination, which was on the other side of the dojo. However, to move just 20, 30 or 40 feet to my right was going to take years of mind and body-busting effort. Did the thought excite, inspire and motivate me? Oh yes, you bet it did!

By the way, the thought of becoming a black belt that first time in the dojo was like standing at the bottom of Everest and looking up with no climbing experience. In truth, that's how it felt to me. Now I am able to look back at my journey and my learning and unpack it in such a way that I can share this amazing system to success with you.

So, let's kick off this process by understanding the criteria of a goal. It's said by many motivational speakers that a goal must be made up of certain things. Things that stimulate emotion. There are lots of acronyms out there with one of the most famous being the S.M.A.R.T. goal, brought about by author and entrepreneur, Professor George T Duran. S.M.A.R.T. stands for Specific, Measurable, Achievable, Relevant and Time-bound.

I don't think anyone can argue with this application for setting what I class as objectives. But, in my opinion, it can't be applied in the same way to inspirational, impactful life-changing goals.

Therefore, I'm going to provide you with my version. This is the formula that will enable you to achieve something very special indeed. I have aptly named it...

G.E.N.E.S.I.S.

The GENESIS goal-setting system, for me, is the essence of what a goal design should look like. Genesis means 'the origin or formation of something', which is the perfect definition of this system. Although, I will add the word 'special' so it becomes 'the origin of something special'. Something visionary, something creative, something strategic and something dynamic.

Here is G.E.N.E.S.I.S.

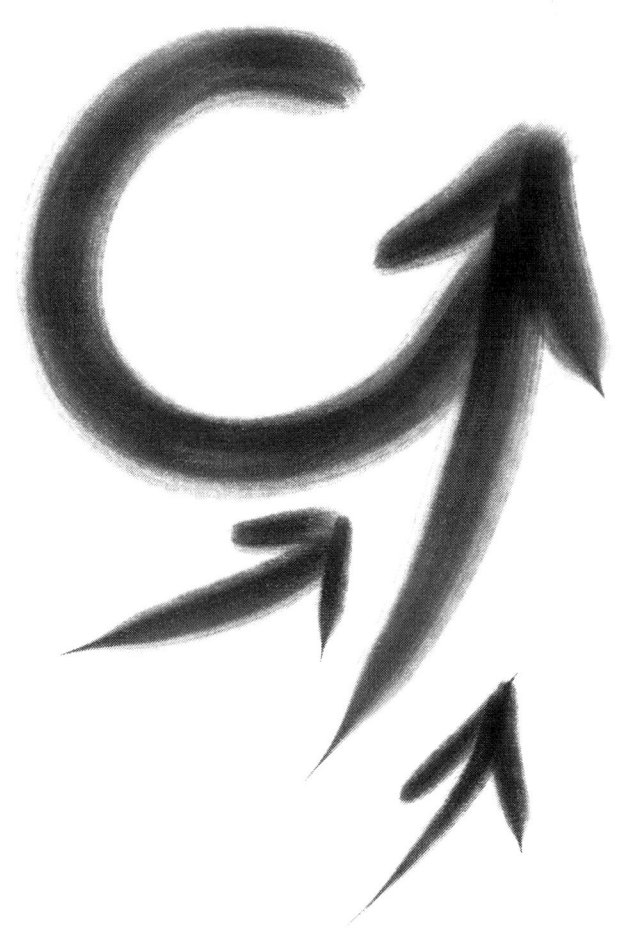

GOOSEBUMPS:

Goosebumps occur as a result of strong emotion, such as fear or shock. They also appear when you're cold. However, they tend to materialise when witnessing an amazing feat or something incredibly inspiring. I want your goal to be so inspirational, so meaningful, it will make your hair stand on end when you think about it. Does it give you goosebumps?

EXTENT:

To what extent are you willing to go to reach your goal? How far can you stretch yourself? To create change in life, we must change. That's the difficult part. Are you prepared to stick it out? Don't limit the range or size of your goals.

NARRATIVE:

What does the goal look like? Believe it, visualise it. Design the narrative based around this. What is the meaning and purpose behind it? Why is the goal so important? What's the bigger picture? What impact will this have on you and the lives of others? It's time to get creative and use your imagination, which has been said to be our greatest skill. What can we dream up? In the words of the American self-help author Napoleon Hill, 'A goal is a dream with a deadline.' Dream big, my readers.

EDIT:

You have the narrative in place; the picture of the goal and the level of impact it could achieve. Now go over it one more time, one last edit. Refine it and define it and now shine it up to be the most inspirational image you can dream up. Give it a name, and invent a goal statement that perfectly depicts the goal. This must inspire you every time you say it out loud or think about it. Your response to this will take you back to the G in the GENESIS model; goosebumps. This part gives the brain what it craves… clarity. Clarity in goal setting is the magic ingredient, we want the clearest, most impactful picture possible. You must work hard at this point to take the vision to another level.

Let me share a short, but moving, true story of the naming of a goal. This is what crystallising a goal can mean. It relates to a client who suffered with a serious mental health issue. In his fifties, he was, and still is, a hugely successful man, but he believed his mental health struggles started some ten years before we met, following the passing of his dearly loved mother. He described his life from then on, and at the point when we met, as being in 'an incredibly dark place'. While my client knew he had been unwell for several years, he admitted that he had spent the past three years trying to 'fix himself' but to no avail. He rated most areas of his life between one and three out of ten, including his self-esteem, confidence, sleep and social capability levels.

I believe our meeting was a great example of fate taking a hand. I had seen him at the gym at few times previously and, in passing, I simply asked, 'How are you?' That opened up a conversation during which he shared with me that he was in a bad way and needed help. Those were his exact words.

Our paths first crossed on a Monday and he agreed to meet me later that week for coaching. At the start of our first session, I said to him, 'It's OK – you're in safe hands now,' and he began to cry. I watched this 6ft 1', strong, professionally successful man, break down in front of me.

At this point, my client knew he needed to take time off work. He'd already been prescribed the maximum quantity of antidepressant drugs and still he couldn't get the darkness to lift. Along our coaching journey I discovered he was also on blood pressure tablets, and he had been for years. During one session I asked what it would feel like to come off his blood pressure and antidepressant medication? He said, 'That would be utopia, Phil!' So his goal statement became one word; 'utopia'.

The coaching process, including the fixing, development and strengthening of his inner fortress paid huge dividends. After months of working together, he was signed off by the doctor to return to work and, little by little, he came off the antidepressants under the guidance of his GP. The darkness had started to lift. One day, out of the blue, I received a text from him. It contained just one word: 'utopia!' He was finally free from all medication including his blood pressure tablets.

This client is another amazing and inspirational example of what people can discover within themselves and then use it to take action. It's all there inside you – a wealth of innate wonders, I promise.

Is it easy to climb Everest? NO! Is it possible? YES!

STRATEGY:
You have your vision, now it's time to plan the mission. You have a crystal-

clear goal and recognise its value and the impact it's going to have. Now it's time to get strategic and plot out the goal journey. This is your action plan. What's the first thing you are going to do? Then the next and the next… Start to drop in a timeline with some key points of reference as illustrated by the line of coloured belts in karate. Be specific and commit to it. Remember small steps; small but important wins along the way are critical.

IMPLEMENTATION:
You have all the dreams and goals in your head and on paper, but now it's about action. The doing part of the goal. The wonderful thing about implementation is that it makes you feel confident and competent. You have designed an inspirational goal. You have painstakingly thought it through and devised an achievable and measurable process to reach it. Design a goal affirmation and shout it out loud. It will have so much power and give you goosebumps. The positive effect of affirmations is also backed up by science. They help to cement your commitment and self-belief. You must start with your goals, then add your affirmation to them and not the other way round. Just make sure each one is expressed in the present tense, for example it could contain some of your core values that will take you to your goal. 'I am resilient' or 'I am proud of myself, I am grateful for…' If you feel unstoppable then say 'I am unstoppable!' What does this provide you with? The answer is a big smile, real confidence and the ability to spend more time in the moment. Stick to the strategy, stay with the process and enjoy your life changes along the way.

SUCCESS:
Any goal-setting process should include a celebration of success. Success means something different to everyone, therefore you have to define it yourself. It is described as 'the accomplishment of an aim or purpose'. It's the opposite of failure. When working with my clients I talk about reaching a goal as taking them to the starting line not the finish line. Why should the journey stop when you have the rest of your life in front of you? You can use energy from this achievement to fuel more goals. Practising gratitude is a beautiful way to celebrate your success and share it with those in your life.

The English poet William Blake said, '*What is now proved was once only imagined.'* Think about that for a moment please.

So let's delve a little more into the power of the imagination for a second. A study by Erin M. Shackell and Lionel G. Standing, of Bishop's University, revealed that you may be able to make nearly identical gains in strength and fitness without lifting a finger! The study measured the strength gains in three different groups of people. The first group did nothing outside their usual routine. The second group was put through two weeks of highly focussed strength training for one specific muscle, three times a week. The third group listened to audio CDs that guided them to imagine themselves going through the same workout as the exercising group, three times a week.

The results were mind-blowing. The control group, who didn't do anything, saw no gains in strength. The exercise group, who trained three times a week, saw a 28% gain in strength. No big surprises there. However, the group who did not exercise, but rather thought about exercising, experienced nearly the same gains in strength as the exercise group achieving 24%. Yes, you read that right! The group that visualised exercise got nearly the same benefit as the group that actually worked-out.

You will, no doubt, be familiar with the saying 'seeing is believing', but author and philosopher Bob Proctor talks about this in reverse. He states, *'believing comes first then the seeing next'.* He is right, of course, we need that confidence to help define the mental picture. Without true inner belief you can forget about achieving any goals. Just reread that last sentence a few more times – it is so true.

You have to *believe* it's possible. Setting goals that are off the belief spectrum will create a reverse reaction. They will turn into burdens and demotivate you, not inspire you. Work within that spectrum but make it really challenging at the far end – the life-changing part of the scale. Also note, the word 'hopeful' never works in the goal-setting process. I worked with a small business as a coach and consultant and banned this word from everyday communications. I noticed early in the relationship that everyone used this word. 'Yes, hopefully'; 'hopefully, we'll hit the completion date'; 'hopefully, I'll get this done today'. I couldn't believe what I was hearing. An air traffic controller does not possess the word 'hopefully' in his vocabulary, so we removed this non-committal type of language from their business communications dictionary and focussed on greater clarity and commitment across everything they did. Being hopeful will not change anything – believing will.

The seeing and believing parts are critical because when fused together they create immense power, but you will achieve nothing without the 'doing' part of the process. As they say – 'actions speak louder than words.'

In the dojo, the ultimate goal is a route, travelling down the line to this magical space where the black belts hang out. You can see it and sense it. It's your unique and personal journey.

In his book, *Atomic Habits,* James Clear says that the most powerful of all sensory abilities in a human being is vision and half of the brain's resources are used on vision. He goes on to say, '*What you see influences what you do.*'

I must share with you one of my experiences regarding visualisation. In karate we practise mastering three disciplines – *kihon* (basic moves, blocks, punches and stances), *kumite* (fighting) and *kata* (a series of moves practised to perfection that represent a sequence of defence and attacks). The moves within a particular *kata* (and there are many), can range from twenty to sixty.

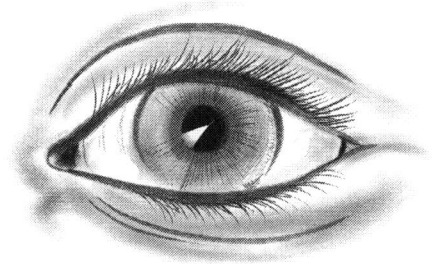

As is the case for many karate students, my *kata* was by far my weakest discipline. I used to hide at the back of the class when *katas* were called and suffered unreserved humiliation when I got them wrong in front of the class.

I became so fed up with this negative mindset towards kata, I set out to make it a strength. I practised relentlessly my eight katas, time and time again. I watched videos of masters executing the moves to precision and, in my mind, perfection. But this is the point I want to make. I practised them everywhere I could, at home, on holiday, in the garden, in my office – I even practised them all in the bath! Yes, in the bath, I 'visualised' them and one in particular called Bassai Dai. It's the *kata* you need to perfect to pass your black belt exam and it has forty-two movements.

Due to this change in mindset, I reached a level that meant I could ask my sensei to call any *kata,* after a training session, and I would go on to nail it. It became a strength not a weakness and I used visualisation as a means to reach a different level of success, but more importantly a different mindset.

So, that example happened inside the dojo. However, when we step outside the world of karate, the goal-setting process must start with exactly the same approach – indisputable belief, vision, visibility and visualisation. Fire up your imagination, let it take you to a new destination and begin to build that mental picture of what the goal looks like.

The process is so simple yet so clever. You are staring at a roadmap of the onward journey, the way, as well as the end goal. It's right in front of your eyes, you are surrounded by it, you can feel it emotionally and spiritually, which becomes more intense the further down the line of the goal you travel.

Next you must work on the quality of the mental goal image by scanning it in your mind until it develops many layers of authenticity and reality. It almost transforms into a physical image, like a 3D picture or a 3D model whereby it has 360-degree visibility.

Then further refining and unpacking is needed. Keep at it. You now have the vision, this is the *'what'* part of the process; what the goal looks like. Now it's time for the *'why'*. Why is the goal important to you? Why is this so valuable, hence life-changing? Then comes the *'who'*. Who is going to benefit from this goal? Describe the impact achieving this will have on your life and 'who else' inside and outside of your world.

I'm going to refine this process a little further – please take note, it's hugely important. Write your goals down. It makes a colossal difference to the probability of you achieving them and there is science to support this. Vividly describing goals in writing is heavily related with goal success. A Harvard business study revealed some extremely interesting statistics relating to goal setting. It found that the 14% of people who have goals are ten times more successful than those without goals. Now keep this in mind. The 3% with written goals were three times more successful that the 14%. That makes the 3% thirty times more successful than people without goals.

Writing things down, or journaling as it is called, provides a deeper sensory experience. It helps you to understand your goals more clearly. It improves memory, it's visual too and conserves the brain's energy as it doesn't need to hold on to the data anymore. It works – trust me!

My clients often hear me say, 'But can you really see the goal? Can you feel it? Can you touch it? Is it real? Describe it in detail, I want to feel it, too. Are the goosebumps happening?' If they answer, 'yes' to those questions then that's magnificent! Then it's time to work on the *'how and when'*. How are we going to get there? How will the journey unfold? What is the timeline?

We now have the goal, it's in widescreen 3D and it's inspirational. We have established it's conceivable and achievable no matter how challenging. So, to use a well-used and meaningful coaching term, what's next?

The answer is – setting the process, the strategy. It's time to devise the plan, the route, the way to reach the goal. This is why the karate process is the perfect analogy for goal setting.

As you now know, the first step to black is to white belt then to orange. It's a strategic stepping stone, it's deliberate and is made up of many layers of smaller requirements for you to complete to place you in the perfect position to move on to the next step, in this case it's the red belt. Tiny steps are taken in order to reach the ultimate goal.

Most importantly, the process has its own inbuilt measurement system. The goal journey must be measurable. If it's not, then how do you know where in the process you are? Measurement is critical for the process to work. In karate we measure our progress by status, the colour of our belt, but this could be broken down further by adding in a timeline and milestones within each belt journey.

I did one of my presentations, called 'The Gateway to Greater Mental Fitness', for an insurance institution in the City of London. When describing the goal-setting process, I used a slide showing this striking but very old, impassable bridge built over a stunning river. It's such a beautiful image. I said the goal is the other side of the river and we have to build a new bridge, bit by bit, stone by stone, stage by stage, to reach the other side. This is the goal-setting process. By showing the audience the picture – it simply helped them visualise the journey and the end goal.

Have you heard of *kaizen*? It's a Japanese term for 'change for the better' or 'continuous improvement'. It's a philosophy of small improvements over time to produce big results. It was adapted and used in business, especially manufacturing. Big goals sometimes get lost and abandoned but if you break them down into small parts and produce small changes then huge future impacts can be revealed. It's like the 1% rule. Improving by 1% a day makes you thirty-seven times better after a year. That's what the maths says.

When I was studying brain-based coaching communications with the NeuroLeadership Institute, I discovered an interesting process they used for establishing a goal. It's referenced as mining, refining, defining and shining. *'Mining'* is a metaphor for uncovering areas of need from a client's world that they might require some help with. *'Refining'* is creating a series of inspiring goals that could potentially be combined in some way. Once this is done then the *'defining'* process begins with setting clear, inspiring, challenging and visionary primary goals within the areas of need established by the mining and refining elements. These goals are verified by creating goal statements with a metric of measurement included.

Then the goals are *'shined'*, turning into precious jewels of life by completing a series of questions such as: what are the three key emotions that describe how you feel when you reach your goal? If your goal was a slogan on your T-shirt, what would it say? And how can we transform this goal, so it inspires you every time you say it?

This brain-based process ensures the journey is solution-focussed but challenging to create new thinking and personal growth, always looking forward, creating positivity and motivation. Our brains tend to zone into problems as this is our default mode. Setting goals blows this mindset away and, in particular, when looking at performance. This entire system from white to black belt translates into achieving a life of optimal performance.

I am convinced that if you drop into the process of the six magical pillars underpinning this book – honesty, trust, commitment, discipline, perseverance and accountability, whatever your goal, small or large, developmental or transformational, you will achieve it.

Being a student of mindfulness, I spent some time wrestling with goal setting. As you will learn when you reach the green belt syllabus, mindfulness is about spending as much time as you can in the present moment, not dwelling on the past nor concerning yourself with the future. Mindfulness is about paying attention to the here and now with acceptance but without judgement. Eckhart Tolle, a spiritual teacher and bestselling author says, *'Most of us are here but our minds are in the future.'* The only place we can ever be is here, so how does goal setting fit in to a mindful way of living?

The answer is this. Once the goal has been established. Then it's all about the path, the way to reach it – the process. Remember *kaizen,* if the pathway is clear and concise and the signposts, like the coloured belts, are all pointing towards your destination then you can relax, forget about the goal and just enjoy the journey, living in the here and now, moment-by-moment, step by step. It's both beautiful and remarkable, as you don't have to be still or stationary to be present, you can be moving – flowing like water.

Bruce Lee said, *'Be like water. Water has no shape, and it becomes whatever it is poured in to be it a cup, a bottle or a teapot.' 'Be formless,'* he says. My view as to what he meant by that is you need to change, adapt and grow when facing certain situations. He goes on to say that no matter how hard he punched or struck water he couldn't hurt it. It appears weak yet can cut through the hardest substance in the world. It needs to be moving, though. Think about it, this clear, neutral fluid that we drink and wash with has the power to cut through mountain ranges when it's moving. As soon as it stops moving what happens? It becomes stagnant and disappears. 'Be like water', my friend. That's just so beautiful.

Set yourself astonishing goals with life-changing outcomes. Don't go for green, purple or brown belt goals, go for black and beyond and create them using the GENESIS system.

'When it is obvious that the goals cannot be reached, don't adjust the goals, adjust the action steps.' ~ CONFUCIUS

RED BELT GRADING WARM-UP:

My definition of a goal is: 'A goal is an inspirational challenge outside the zone of comfort that when accomplished impacts life in a truly positive way.'

The brain loves clarity and certainty and there is no better way to provide this than by adopting a goal-setting mindset. It creates a certain power and helps destroy the waves of uncertainty life challenges us with. Convert your dreams into goals, designing what your life could look like. Don't be afraid to stretch yourself out of that area of mental safety, you will be surprised what you can achieve.

In this syllabus, we zoned into the clear process used in karate as an example and analogy of how a goal-setting process should be designed. There should be clear visibility, motivation, stretching and pushing limits. Small steps bring huge results with a journey full of wins and accomplishments.

We used my GENESIS model to help drive the goal to that special place whereby your life and others are impacted by its success. However, success can only be guaranteed when applying the six pillars of the way to the process.

HONESTY – what does the outcome and impact truly look like? Remember the why?

TRUST – have faith. Once you have designed the goal and the goal journey you must trust the process and back yourself, believe in yourself. Belief is key to success.

COMMITMENT – it's simple, without 100% of this element the process fails.

DISCIPLINE – your goal will incorporate changes, new ways, new routines and doing new things. Discipline creates new habits by repeating the drills, exercises or routines.

PERSEVERANCE – creating any change in life is by no means easy. We are met with obstacles that test us both from our inner and outer worlds. Never give up and always persevere. Keep adapting, keep moving. You will get there. You will achieve. 'Be like water.'

ACCOUNTABILITY – own your goal. Either make it the world's best kept secret keeping your accountability a private affair or, better still, tell the world what it is, what it looks like and the impact it's going to have. Share it with everyone you come into contact with. This forces accountability as you have to own it from then on. This is so important; you must own the goal with a smile and a positive attitude.

RED BELT GRADING

1. Read 'The Man in the Glass' again.

2. Go to your journal – your 'book of life' – and revise and reflect on what you have entered so far. Review your belief system. Your core values, gratitude and so on. This should get the positive neurochemistry flowing.

3. If you have discovered you possess more values along the way then add them to your value system, it grows as you do and vice versa. You must be loyal and committed to the additions, though. Remember 'The Man in the Glass'.

4. Now it's time to design and build goals. Please note that it's goals, plural. The brain needs to be stretched and one goal will be too simplistic for your intelligence. Aim for a minimum of one professional and one personal goal.

5. Read back through the chapter and revisit the process.

6. Construct your goals using the GENESIS model. Aim high and make them as clear and pure as you can.

TIPS TO HELP YOU IDENTIFY YOUR GOALS:

1. If this book was a magic goal genie that would grant you three wishes, what would they be? Remember you must stick to the goal-setting conditions, though. Bow to the book and make the three wishes.
2. Consider setting one goal for each of your life arenas such as, work, family, well-being, personal. Make at least one a 'black belt' goal – stretch yourself.
3. Ask yourself, what do I love doing, what gives me the greatest joy? What can I do to make a difference?
4. Dig deep and go through the mining, refining, defining and shining procedure to find clarity.
5. Take your time. Goal setting is not a one-minute process.
6. You should now have some hugely powerful and precious goals that now require you to build that bridge – the way to reach them. The system is underpinned by the six pillars of the way.
7. Finally, write them down applying strict attention to detail to the goals.

You can do it, I promise you. Be inspired – grasp this opportunity right now. There's no better moment. And if you set up the process skilfully, these small steps will deliver sensational results.

'Our goals can only be reached through the vehicle of a plan, in which we must fervently believe, and upon which we must vigorously act. There is no other route to success.' ~ PABLO PICASSO

Congratulations!
You are now a red belt.
Give yourself a huge pat on the back!
It's a wonderful achievement!

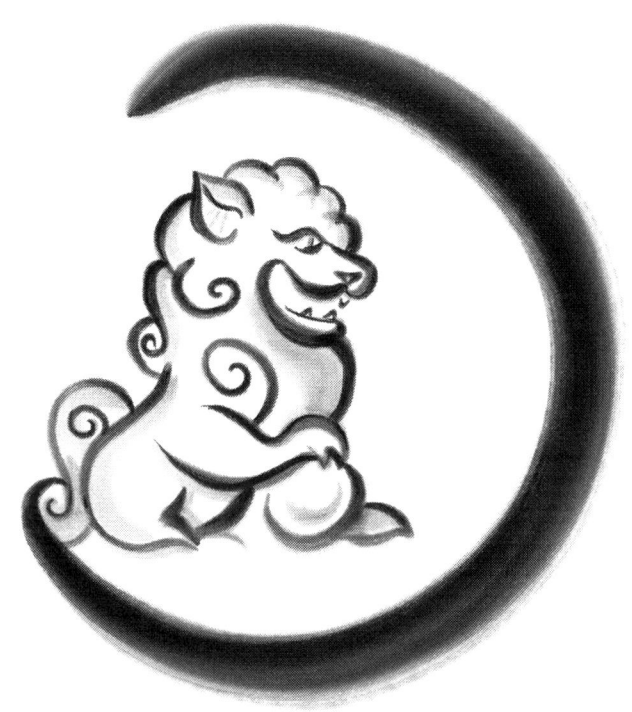

CHAPTER 4
YELLOW BELT
Control and Conquer

'The greatest weapon against stress is our ability to choose one thought over another.' ~ WILLIAM JAMES

It's been said from the outset that this book is a journey to something special. It's your trip of a lifetime. We have acknowledged that we all have a hidden vault of untapped potential and, as we proceed through each grading, we will start to unlock that buried treasure. We have also learned that any success we may achieve starts with thought, or thinking, and our attitude towards personal growth is critical to living a black belt life.

You have acquired six pillars of the way, a life model that must be applied to your own personal adventure and developed into a sound belief structure in order to access self-belief and greater self-esteem. Mental core strength is the platform to build from as, when in place, it provides the opportunity to design some incredible life-changing goals, pulling you outside your comfort zone.

Within the architecture of the way attention to detail plays a massive role. And it's that inner focus, paying close attention to ourselves, that is pivotal at this juncture. We are now going to dive deeper inside.

To achieve yellow belt, in this chapter, we will take self-awareness to new levels and learn to understand more about the brain and the power of the mind when responding to inner and outer challenges and the physiology that occurs. It's important to maintain this self-growth attitude as the more you discover about yourself the more you will become sensitive to what's occurring and why. This brings with it the ability to develop superior emotional control. A greater self-understanding delivers higher confidence levels.

As we move through this grade into the green and then purple belt syllabuses, I will teach you how to respond to, manage and control stress, giving you proven techniques to help you cope with what life throws at you.

SELF-CONTROL

I searched for various definitions and found this one: 'Self-control is the ability to regulate and alter your responses in order to avoid undesirable behaviours, increase desirable ones and achieve long-term goals.' For me, that's just about perfect.

In the dojo we have to become skilled in control to avoid hurting someone else and ourselves, but also to keep focussed and manage our minds and bodies during times of stress. It especially helps us when we meet a highly challenging situation when fighting and/or fatigued. We are trained to keep our emotions in check and not become overwhelmed or angry. Anger is the enemy inside the dojo but when does getting angry have a positive effect outside the dojo? Can you think of a time in your life where anger has ever led to a positive outcome? When has it made you feel good or improved a situation?

Keeping calm, yet maintaining that laser-like focus, is a skill we can all develop. However, we first need to understand what happens to us when we are faced with immensely stressful situations. What physiology actually occurs within us when we activate yet another innate miracle – our survival system. This reaction is sometimes referred to as 'fight or flight'.

I will help you to understand a little more about this astonishing instinctive survival system we all possess. Our fight or flight modes can, literally, keep us alive when we are staring death in the face, but at the same time they can also cause long-term damage.

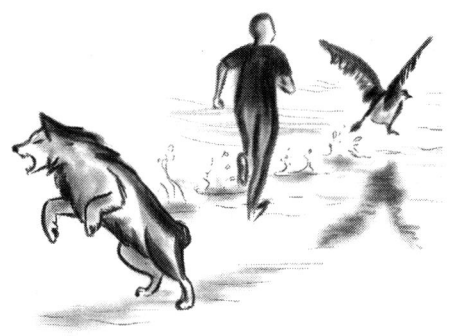

Fight or flight has also been referred to as 'fight, flight, freeze' but, back in the 1920s, a physiologist named Walter Cannon described, what he called, 'the acute stress response'. It's all about how people react to perceived threats.

It's the primitive part of the brain's evolution, whereby the brain developed an automatic response to threats. This neurological early warning system in the brain is called the amygdala. It's an almond-shaped gland situated near the base of the brain and a part of the limbic system which is a cluster of parts that together process and regulate emotions and behaviours as well as other functions. This amazing natural radar scans five times a second for threat or danger.

I have heard the fight or flight response referred to as kill or be killed many times, followed by the analogy of a caveman coming face to face with a sabre-toothed tiger. Anyway, like ours, his brain's primary purpose is to keep him alive, whatever it takes. Therefore, his brain-based threat detection system sets off some neural-alarm bells. And within a second, he has to decide to fight, flee or freeze? Can he win the fight? Is there an escape route or should he freeze, play dead hoping the beast is not interested in him? What are the best odds for survival? He's literally staring death in the face. So, this system is built in to help you survive a true-life threat or danger. That's the good news. We have this incredible system at our disposal that we don't have to consciously activate – it's initiated instantaneously as an automatic reflex.

Now for the bad news…any perceived fear or threat can manifest itself in many other ways and, unfortunately, this can also set off our survival system response, often unnecessarily.

I'm going to provide you with further insight by referring to an incident I happened to find myself in the middle of, that set off my own fight or flight system.

On 27th November 2017, I was in Oxford Street, London, on a shopping trip, as part of my daughter's twentieth birthday celebrations. Accompanying me and my daughter were her mum and boyfriend. I should add that shopping with other people is not my favourite pastime, compounded by the fact it was a Friday. Shopping in central London is bad enough, but on a Friday!

Now let me add a little more drama. We didn't realise until the last minute that it was Black Friday – the Friday following thanksgiving in the United States when many shops have huge sales, opening early and closing late, now common in the UK.

To ramp up the situation to a more serious level, earlier in the year there had been a surge of terrorist incidents in the UK, London in particular, and the national threat level was at the highest.

However, I was outvoted when I suggested rearranging the trip and we travelled into London by train. We started off in Covent Garden in a posh burger restaurant and I attempted to discourage my daughter from visiting Oxford Street, to no avail. I had a bad feeling but wanted my daughter to enjoy her day.

The streets and the shops in Oxford Street were heaving with people, and you could hardly move. The first shop we entered was a massive clothing shop called Zara. I found it a little overwhelming inside and needed to get some air. It was, by now, around 4.30 pm and I decided to take a walk along Oxford Street to Regent Street to see the Christmas lights. I arranged to meet up with the others when they'd finished in Zara.

I left the shop and made my way along the packed pathways. It wasn't long before a police car went past with the lights and sirens in full operation. This is commonplace so I didn't give it another thought. But then another car went past, and another and then a van. At least six police vehicles went past me in the direction I was walking. It occurred to me that this must be a serious incident, however I kept going.

On the approach to Oxford Circus Underground Station, I started to feel anxious. I looked up at the station entrance, and a sign said 'closed due to incident'. At that moment, I heard people shouting and screaming. It was a horrific noise. Then, around the corner from the station came hundreds of people running, yelling, crying, panicking, shouting, 'They've got guns, they've got guns!'

It was a like a wave of people running in terror, in fear of their lives. I appeared to be in the middle of a full-on terrorist incident. Many people swept past me in the chaos. I turned and bolted along with everyone else. In terms of my fight, flight or freeze system it calculated that my best chance of survival was to run, and run fast. I was not going to win a fight against people with guns, standing still was not an option either so it was down to an escape strategy. My rapid response system told me to run! And I did!

I felt like I was running for my life. I was well into my fifties and went from a standing start to a full-on sprint. This is the truth, for maybe ten or twenty seconds I was anticipating getting shot in the back, I was waiting for the sound of gunfire. I was exposed and vulnerable. I wondered if this was it, had my time ran out?

While I was sprinting, I was focussed on two things, my survival and my family a little further down the road. What should I do? Firstly, get to a safe place. I veered off Oxford Street and collided with people running in the opposite direction, screaming, and knocking over those of us travelling the other way. I picked myself up and noticed that the panic had now reached the area I was in, as people in shops and restaurants were anxiously locking their doors and shutters. I turned left again, then right and found myself in a dark alley. I had no idea where I was.

Suddenly, I was alone, but I could still hear police sirens. By now I was hyperventilating. I had hit genuine panic mode. I stopped, tried to control my breath and get my bearings. My mind was confused, and I couldn't gather my composure as much as I tried. With more focus on my breathing, I started to gain mental control. I called my wife and my daughter answered her mobile. I told her to stay in the shop as there was a terrorist attack in progress. She thought I'd been injured because I could not speak properly and the inner terror that I was experiencing transferred to her. I quickly gained more strength and coherence and managed to explain to my daughter's boyfriend where I was, and that I was safe, having then established my location was away from the threat zone. The three of them escaped the shop and came to find me using a sat-nav app on their smartphones. Then we planned our escape route to another area of London. Just after we met, the police completely locked down Oxford Street for a number of hours.

When we were reunited, even after just a few minutes apart, it was very emotional with lots of hugs and tears. But we were safe, at least for the time being – we still had to make it home.

So, I ask you this; what had actually happened to me? Before a karate training session, we go into a well-drilled warm-up that involves lots of stretching and movement to get good blood flow and muscle movement before we start another physically and mentally intense session. But I had gone from a cold standing start into a full-on, flat-out race for survival and didn't feel a thing. I had experienced a perfect example of a fight or flight response to a life-threatening situation. My innate survival mechanism had kicked in.

During those few minutes this is what occurred in my brain and body. As soon as I heard screaming and saw people rushing towards me, the amygdala sent a distress signal to my hypothalamus. This fired up my autonomic nervous system, which includes two other component systems, the sympathetic nervous system and parasympathetic nervous system that play different roles with a fight or flight reaction. An excellent analogy appeared in an article in *Harvard Health* called 'Staying Healthy'. It says the sympathetic nervous system acts like a gas pedal in a car providing a burst of energy to the body, whereas the parasympathetic system functions like a brake. It slows down and calms the body after the danger has passed.

These are the physiological events that then took place in my body in response to the situation:

- An instant message from my hypothalamus was sent to my adrenal glands. They responded by pumping the hormone epinephrine into my blood stream. Epinephrine is also known as adrenaline.
- My heart started beating faster than normal, raising my blood pressure to increase and speed up the blood supply to various areas of my body, providing much-needed extra energy, and boosting strength.
- Blood was instantaneously directed, at speed, to the major muscles in my arms and legs carrying with it the sugars and fats stored within my body that I needed most to fight or flee. My muscles tensed preparing to fight or run.
- Other hormones such as testosterone and cortisol were pumped into my system as well as endorphins to kill any pain.
- My hair stood on end. Ridiculous as it seems, to make me look larger than I am. This is one of many things that we inherited from our ancestors.
- My breathing rapidly increased causing the airways to my lungs to automatically dilate to take in more oxygen to send to the brain, increasing alertness and expelling carbon dioxide more quickly also.
- My pupils dilated to increase peripheral vision, to sharpen up my surroundings and let in more light to help me see better.
- My hearing became more acute.
- The palms of my hands became sweaty as sweating is a natural cooling system to keep the body in prime condition.
- My blood started to thicken with a natural blood coagulant as a precaution to being cut in a fight.
- My mouth went dry, as saliva is part of the digestive system, which slowed down as the energy required to run was redirected to more important areas of need. This is why some people also feel sick.
- My spleen emptied its blood cells into circulation.
- My kidneys stopped urine formation for this brief time, as again this part of my bodily function was not required.
- The colour went from my face, as blood from there was diverted to my brain and major muscles.
- My liver started working overtime to produce more glucose and fats to convert into energy.

I have just described to you in layman's terms what happened to me from the inside out, responding to what I perceived to be a seriously dangerous situation coming at me from the outside in.

When you think about it, you cannot help but gasp at this natural miracle that takes place within a split second. It is something that, along with many other day-to-day bodily functions, thoughts, feelings and emotions, many of us take for granted.

So, as I inferred earlier, this was me coming face to face with the sabre-toothed tiger, a response to a physical and life-threatening situation. By the way the incident was later reported in the media to be a false alarm. But that's another story!

The survival system is present as a short-term explosion of physiological reactions and then it quietly returns to normal after a short while. However, a sensation of fatigue and pain usually follows. It's absolutely incredible what our brains and bodies can do. After just a few minutes my body started to hurt. I went from no pain to shooting pains in my legs. My thighs and calves started to cramp up and my chest tightened. My body felt like it was in shock. It definitely was.

Now, let me share this with you – the brain doesn't know the difference between illusion and reality. I could recreate that event in my mind while lying in bed, creating a psychological threat and start the activation of my survival system again causing adrenaline and cortisol to flood my body.

There are other stories of when the fight or flight or survival system kicks in and people respond with extraordinary strength or speed in response to extreme, unexpected and, usually, life-threatening situations. One of my favourites was the lady in Canada who fought off a 700 lb polar bear to protect her two sons. They all survived.

Moving on from our prehistoric ancestors many of us face psychological threats that emanate from our own thinking in response to certain situations. This response causes us to go into threat mode which, in time, can turn to stress, anxiety and chronic conditions. It has been proven scientifically that the same part of the brain, the anterior cingulate cortex, is affected both from physical pain and a non-physical threat such as being rejected or excluded. I have heard it said that a pain reducing pill, such as a paracetamol, can also reduce emotional pain. To make it clear, pain can be generated by the power of thought. The three fears that trouble so many of us are failure, rejection and fear of the unknown. I can bolt on humiliation as a by-product of failure and rejection, too. These fears are mindset driven, we are not born with them; we develop them over time, creating self-limitations as we do so.

Alan Lokos, a famous American teacher of meditation said, 'Don't believe everything you think, thoughts are just that – thoughts.' What this means, however, is that we have the capability to do something about them! So, we are back to the good news part of this yellow belt syllabus. For example, how did I deal with the fear of humiliating myself in front of a packed dojo on my first training session? And subsequent sessions too? Surely, this is self-made fear, isn't it?

Basically, I battled with my thinking, I went to war with my ego and won! I got out the way of myself and kept turning up and showing up with the right attitude time and time again. Was it challenging? Did I have to search my soul for strength? Yes, but the goal, my exciting and inspirational goal in the form of a black silk belt displaced the fear and won the war against my ego. It was far more powerful than my fear. Susan Jeffers, the American psychologist and author says, *'Feel the fear and do it anyway.'* It's about making yourself accountable. Without realising it, this is exactly what I did. The mind-power we have at our disposal, once we are trained and understand it, is astonishing.

It always starts with thought, thinking patterns, our perception, and the design of our mental pictures. Do you ever overthink situations? So many of us overthink things. Many years ago, I became an expert at it. When I look back, I ask what good did it do? It just caused me stress and many sleepless nights.

But what is stress and how do we control it? Stress can be described as the point at which you feel overcome or unable to cope as a result of pressures that are uncontrollable. The word 'stress' is quite modern when applied to humans. It was previously used as a scientific term in physics, in terms of stress and levers. It's now defined as a state of mental emotion or emotional strain or tension resulting from adverse or demanding circumstances.

So, how do we keep calm and avoid cognitive distortion? Cognitive distortion is a way of thinking that causes people to view reality inaccurately, mostly negatively and irrationally. People catastrophise, try to read other people's minds, blame, dwell, misinterpret, magnify, jump to conclusions and have a tendency to focus on a negative. Does this ring a bell?

For example, my train is delayed, which means I won't make a meeting, that could stop a strategic business deal being closed, then I will lose a blue-chip customer that will result in job losses, me being fired, losing the house because I cannot pay the mortgage, then my wife leaves me with the kids.

That line of thinking lasted a minute or two and I went from a delayed train to being single, without my wife, children and income! Using the train as a metaphor for my mind, I hopped on the train of negativity, the train of cognitive distortion, and it took me to a dark place. I use the train metaphor a great deal in coaching. The train of 'negative thought' comes into the station. Do we get on it or just let it pass through? The correct answer is acknowledge it and let it go. There are many other analogies but for me none better. The more you consciously practise not hopping on that train of negativity, capturing those thoughts and letting them pass with the train, the more expert you will become. You could argue it's train training as well as brain training!

THE POWER OF THE MIND

Experts believe we have between 60,000 and 80,000 thoughts a day of which 80% are negative and most are repetitive. Do we ever overthink with positive outcomes? No, we overthink ourselves into negativity and, potentially, a fight or flight physiological response. Some of this is not actually your fault – it's simply your brain and how it functions. It takes less energy to focus on a problem than to find a solution, and that's why we tend to overthink a problem; it's easier for the brain.

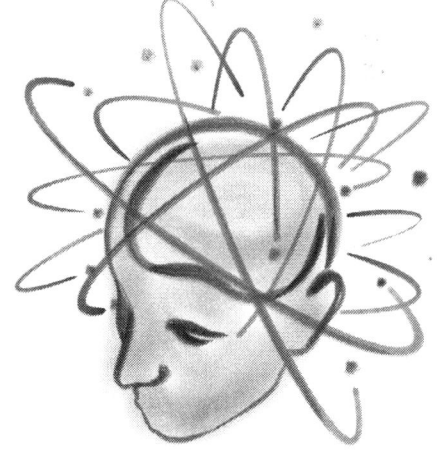

So, now I'm going to flip this conundrum by using the previously mentioned, staggering power of the mind, this time to help us and not harm us.

Your mind can be an amazing healing tool given the opportunity. There is no better example of the power of the mind than the placebo effect. This is when the mind tricks you into thinking that a fake treatment to an illness or symptom can produce healing results and, in some cases, imitate the effects of actual medical treatments. A placebo is administered in the form of a sugar pill or an injection, which is normally saline.

The placebo effect has been found to positively impact people that suffer with depression and anxiety. The power lies with the expectation of the person taking it, which is usually a positive expectation. Amazingly, this affects the same part of the brain that is targeted by antidepressant drugs.

Placebos have been used successfully for management of chronic pain, irritable bowel syndrome (IBS) and even to reduce the symptoms of Parkinson's disease. Although not fully understood, one explanation is that when taking a placebo our minds believe we are being healed, which triggers a release of endorphins, our feel-good chemical, which has a structure similar to morphine and acts as the brain's natural painkiller.

There are many case studies regarding the use of a placebo. One which I found interesting was an experiment conducted by Derren Brown, the illusionist. He named it 'Fear and Faith', a title I love.

Derren set up a fake pharmaceutical company, which he claimed had developed a drug named Rumyodin that inhibited fear. The drug was actually a sugar pill. During this incredibly realistic stage hoax, using professional actors as doctors and lab technicians, Derren got together a group of people suffering with various fears such as heights, social confidence, singing in public and so on. Alongside this, he faked clinical trials promoting Rumyodin to other groups that suffered from allergies, skin disorders and smokers who wanted to quit the habit. The results were staggering. Even when Derren revealed that Rumyodin was in fact an anagram of 'your mind', many of his subjects responded excitedly and positively, as they realised, they themselves had actually defeated their fears and habits purely through the power of belief, without the aid of a drug. They had overcome their fears.

On this unique, but challenging journey, with your belief system in place from your orange belt education, this chapter shows that you have the resources within you to affect huge change using a major life-changing tool. Belief. Belief has the power to change your life on its own but it also helps you to unlock resilience and perseverance, which are magnificent qualities and determine the quality of our lives.

Belief forms your reality, therefore, when you actively don't believe something, it becomes your reality. If you can develop true self-belief you will always find the tools to support it. As we have already established in the orange and red belt syllabuses, our beliefs determine the quality of our lives. And what does belief affect? Yes, our behaviour.

What about this for a story.

I watched Tom Bilyeu, the co-founder of the billion-dollar brand Quest Nutrition and host of *Impact Theory,* interview Trevor Moawad, a famous mental conditioning coach. This is the story he told. It's not quite word for word, but it's sensational.

Trevor Moawad relayed a story about one of the most successful magazine entrepreneurs in the world. The man was failing at high school and struggled growing up. He was raised by a single mum in Midwest America. He promised his mother he'd take the SAT test, the standard test taken by everyone in the USA. It's split in two parts with Maths and English with a total possible score of 800 for each part equating to 1600. He didn't expect to get a good score. He took the test and his score came back. He got an amazing score of 1480 out of 1600 on the SAT. His mother, knowing her kid, asked, 'Did you cheat?' He promised her he hadn't.

In his senior year he realised he was smarter than he thought and decided to attend classes. He stopped hanging out with his old crowd. His teachers and peers seemed to notice the change and began to think that they had missed something about him previously, perhaps, and so they started treating him differently.

He graduated, attended community college, went on to Wichita State, and eventually to a top Ivy League school. He then went on to become an incredibly successful magazine entrepreneur.

You think, he's smart. He just needed the standardised test to unlock his potential and realise he had some key skills he hadn't before noticed. No. This isn't the story. What comes next is the important part.

Twelve years later, the man received a letter in the mail from Princeton, New Jersey. It turns out the SAT board periodically reviews their test taking procedures and policies. He was one of thirteen people sent the wrong SAT score. His actual score was 740.

People say his whole life changed when he got the 1480. What really happened is his behaviour changed. He started acting like a person with a score of 1480 and started doing what someone with a result like that does.

Trevor says language is powerful, but your behaviour is way ahead of your success. The lesson is, in addition to language, how you feel about the past shouldn't determine who you are in the future.

The man believed he was a 1480 and the behaved like a 1480. Isn't that inspirational?

When I heard this story it ratified my theory. I often say to students getting close to their black belt grading, it's time to start behaving like a black belt. Act like a black belt, believe you're a black belt!

In the dojo we are trained to be relaxed in body but focussed mentally. We spend our time in the moment, living life in real time and not dwelling on the past nor thinking about the future. It's moment-to-moment awareness in its purity.

As a white belt we are trained to empty our cup of mental noise before we enter the place of the way, with the aim of leaving our stress and any negativity outside. Now I understand why I felt so refreshed and alive when I bowed and left the dojo after training. It could be after a body-busting training session or teaching as an instructor, but the feeling was and still is exactly the same.

One of the most noticeable things for me, as I started my journey through the grades, was how black belts could turn on and off their laser-like focus like a light switch. When the shift occurred, their eyes transformed to an ice-cold intensity. For me it seemed extraordinary, and I wanted to be able to do it. It was so intimidating. I became really curious to find where this superpower came from. Does everyone acquire this skill? Does it develop over time? Will I get it?

What was actually occurring with these guys when they called upon this superpower? I believe they were in a state of high concentration awareness (HCA), a zone of peak state performance, dialled into while simultaneously being relaxed. This has also been referred to as a state of 'flow', almost like a trance. In his book, *Flow: The Psychology of Optimal Experience,* Mihaly Csikszentmihalyi, a Hungarian-American psychologist, delves into the experience of a mental state when people are so involved nothing else seems to matter. In the book he says, *'Flow is the optimal state of intrinsic motivation where the person is fully immersed in what they are doing.'* I'm sure we can all look back at a time when we experienced 'flow'.

It's happened to me a number of times and it's fair to say that I didn't know what was occurring within me and outside of me too, I just rode the wave. It happened during my black belt exam and, on occasion, on the cricket field, both when batting and bowling. It was as if I was in a state of Zen, totally relaxed while my senses, reactions and coordination were electric. I felt indestructible with a bat or ball in my hand when experiencing this state of mind. I tapped into my skillsets, unlocking my true potential and capabilities while maintaining a mind absent of thought. Literally no conscious thinking would take place, you just let all the learning and preparation that has taken place over the years work instinctively. In a nutshell, you are getting yourself out of the way.

I practised until it became a subconscious action. My karate training ramped up to four or five times a week. I couldn't get enough of it. I just wanted to improve more and more, day by day, until the superpower arrived.

Can you imagine how helpful this superpower can be for public speaking or delivering high-level presentations or just producing day-to-day high-quality work whatever your job. Paying attention and focussing with deep layers of detail without being distracted is such an incredible asset. In karate when facing an opponent, we tune into their eyes, never leaving them. The eyes give away so much. It's taking the saying 'the eyes are the window to the soul' to another level of intensity. Your opponent is constantly trying to distract you with the intention of landing a kick or a punch, either to score a point or much worse in full contact.

In coaching, paying full attention to the client is the first rule of engagement. I refer to it as 'paying attention with intention'. In an interview, I was once asked what my clients gained from me. My answer was 'everything'. From the moment I'm with them to the moment we separate, nothing else exists in my life. They get my soul, my undivided attention and every ounce of my passion to help them achieve their goals. My intention helped me develop my attention resulting in becoming skilled at listening to others, an essential skill needed for my work but something many of us could improve on as people, partners and leaders. Being able to listen without distraction, emotionally committing to a person or a group, and being in the moment, the now, is one of the most precious life tools one can display as a human being.

At work we are battered with many subliminal blows raining down on us in the form of distractions. They are everywhere. An online article published by Workplace Trends called 'How much time do you lose to distractions?' says that the long list of office distractions account for 2.1 hours a day in loss of productivity and that employees spend an average of just eleven minutes on a project before being distracted. Worse still, it takes them twenty-five minutes to regain mental focus back to the original task. They ask the question, 'How do we find a way to reduce all these distractions and make the most of the time available?' I love the response. 'Identify your weapons of mass distraction!' Meaning, your devices, outside noise, in-your-head noise and untidiness also. Basically, shifting focus backwards and forwards takes energy, especially when working on a new task that requires full-on brain power, so you start to use up those valuable energy resources.

Distractions can cause more damage too, affecting the overall quality of your work by less time spent on creative, positive and productive thinking. They can cause you to forget great ideas and insights, which can be immensely frustrating.

One of the obvious ways to reduce distraction is removing all communication devices from your area of work. The brain prefers to focus on things right in front of you because it requires less effort. In his book 'Your Brain at Work', David Rock says that allowing yourself to be distracted is like stopping pain to enjoy a mild pleasure, it's too difficult to resist.

Blocking out distractions is one of the best methods to improve mental performance. But the sorts of distractions that we've covered so far are extrinsic distractions – so what about intrinsic distractions?

Can we control our inner disruptions, the wandering mind? Of course, we can, but yet again this requires a lot of practice, patience and discipline. I have already referenced and will continue to repeat many times, you don't 'get' a black belt you become one. You train and train, you practise moves thousands of times, you execute detailed preparation and then repetition, you refine and hone your awareness and attention skills, until one day something happens, the shift occurs. It happened to me, and I can still turn my focus on and off like a tap. It's an amazing feeling and you can have this, too.

In the dojo, a spaced repetition technique is used. This system works by spacing your learning, giving your brain more time to digest it and create new, deeper embedded wiring for long-term memory, allowing you to complete things automatically without consciously thinking about them. I use this technique in my coaching practice sometimes, apologising for repeating myself or relentlessly reviewing past moments of learning and agreed actions.

As a kid, I played cricket in front of my house and with windows left and right of me I could only hit the ball straight to score. As I grew older I developed into an expert at this and became renowned in my circle of cricket as someone who played textbook straight. This was without one minute of coaching, just playing with my friends and hitting the ball thousands of times in one direction. The more we practise, the more skills and capabilities are stored, which allows our cup to be filled with new learning.

In karate we practise what we call 'combinations'. These can range from two to sometimes six moves to take out an opponent. To become incredibly skilled at a combination we start by practising each move individually to perfect it, then add another, then another and so on until it becomes a seamless combination delivered with speed and precise accuracy. Please do not see this as multitasking, it's paying attention to, and learning, one thing at a time and putting it together to make a system. Multitasking is a myth. We all believe we can multitask. We can't – at least not consciously.

The truth is none of us can actually multitask to high levels of mental performance. For a start, we can only focus on one conscious task at a time. If you try to do two, I'm afraid attention is like a pie, each task will get half each. You will dilute your focus by 50% on each task. This, in turn, uses up more energy and results in lesser quality and more mistakes, a real drop in performance. The only way to do two mental tasks quickly at 100% is to do them one at a time.

You must all have driven to a destination you know with a friend or family member in the car, chatting comfortably all the way there. Now think about when you have had the same person in the car but you're driving to a location you've never been to before. Is the conversation and experience the same? It won't be! That's why when we are lost, we find ourselves turning the volume down on the radio. Constantly splitting focus from one thing to another creates mental exhaustion and can sometimes activate the fight or flight system by being on constant alert.

We can only do this if the things we are doing are already embedded into our subconscious memory, our autopilot and, therefore, do not require the part of our brain called the Prefrontal Cortex (PFC), where our conscious real-time memory and decision-making exists.

The PFC is sometimes referred to as the executive function of the brain or the 'CEO' as it is responsible for high-level cognitive functions.

The cortex is a layer that covers the brain a tenth of an inch thick. The PFC, part of the cortex, is positioned behind your forehead, is about 5% of the brain's volume and is one of the newest evolutionary additions to the brain. Roles of the PFC include our ability to think consciously, planning, choosing, judgement, anticipation and the hugely significant function of goal setting. Conscious decision-making is the job of the PFC and determining what is good and bad.

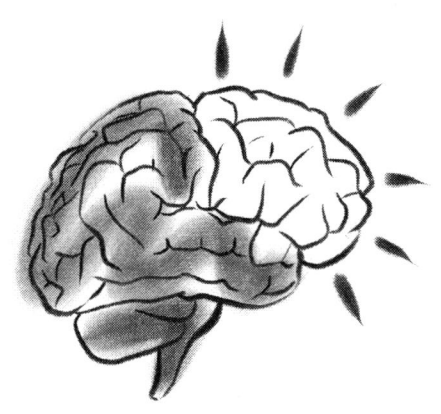

Our PFC is a real-time processing machine and deals with all incoming information from the outside, filtering the flood of data, sending it to various parts of the brain to be actioned.

Conscious thinking saps energy so, like a battery, the PFC gets drained and tired and needs rest, decluttering and recharging. Therefore, some downtime away from mental commotion and a good night of well-hydrated sleep is the best recharging system available to produce that brain sharpness we all look for.

Amy Arnsten, a professor in neurobiology who spent years studying this part of the brain, says 'the PFC holds the contents of your mind at any one point' so you can see why we get tired even without rigorous physical activity.

High-level functions at work will take more out of the PFC so its energy and performance need to be used wisely. Again, we can treat it like a battery and plan and prioritise our levels of engagement for those times we will need our PFC operating at its best. I know it's obvious to say this but the end of a tough day would not be the best time to execute a high-level strategic presentation to your executive team followed by a Q&A! Ask yourself this. Will I be at my sharpest and smartest? The answer is no.

When the PFC is in need of a recharge you could experience a number of feelings such as laziness, lethargy, lack of focus, forgetfulness, negative thinking and over-emotional responses. You will also be distracted easily.

The opposite occurs when it's fired up and full of energy. You will find more clarity with planning, be able to concentrate and have a good sense of self-awareness.

So, apply this learning to your day at work and start to unravel when you feel at your best, when you are struggling and looking for yet another espresso to keep you going. You will discover a window of optimum performance and be able to adjust, modify and prioritise your daily tasks in line with your performance window, thus improving your overall effectiveness and productivity and reducing stress levels. It's planning with your brain in mind! Under stress it doesn't perform well as energy is diverted to other parts of the brain to deal with the issue.

We must be relentless in the pursuit of personal growth, and repetition creates the strongest learning, enabling you to make lasting changes in your brain both physically and mentally. If you think about it, essentially a belief is a thought that has been thought multiple times. How fantastic to know that you can alter your belief system, which will, in turn, change your life. This is why visualisation and affirmations are so powerful. We need the power of our mind and imagination, and we need to vocalise our strength and purpose, as by doing this it becomes much more powerful and really hooks into our subconscious. Let me share a story with you about an affirmation.

I had a client who approached me about his self-discipline. A guy in his mid-forties with a successful career in insurance and a love of sport. He said he had a weight and fitness problem, and it was down to his lack of discipline.

I thought we'd made a good start to the process as the client felt he'd identified an issue. After a few coaching sessions, whereby my client openly talked about his weight issue, describing it as being in his 'number three wardrobe', we ascertained that his goal was to lose enough weight to open up wardrobe two and then wardrobe one.

These goals were very achievable, inspirational and easily measurable as the scales told the story. What transpired over the coaching journey was that the issue went far deeper than weight and self-discipline. This client was destroyed on the inside!

This is what we unpacked over time:

- He had little or no self-esteem and self-confidence.
- He didn't like his reflection in a mirror inside and out.
- His boss for over three years was simply a bully and my client had suffered greatly from psychological intimidation, and it had taken its toll.
- He had come out of two serious relationships, including one marriage, that had a profound effect on his self-esteem, which he rated, at most, as three out of ten.
- He was overweight for sure, but the issue went far deeper than that.
- He felt that he had missed the opportunity for a meaningful and lasting relationship and the thought of having children was just that, a thought with absolutely no substance whatsoever.
- He suffered with procrastination and huge amounts of negative self-talk. His favourite saying was, 'That's just typical of me to find a negative in something – that's what I always do.'
- And most of all, he could not visualise ever being in love again. This wasn't even a dream anymore; he had just dismissed it from all possibility.

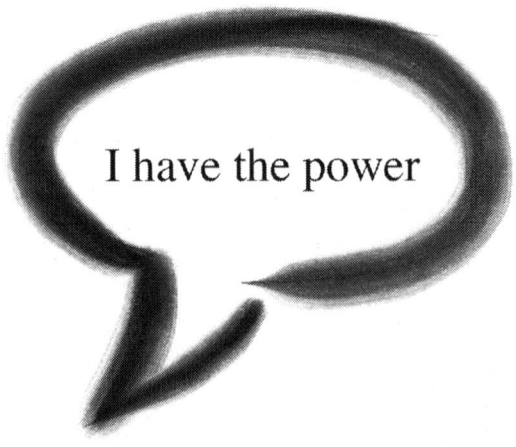

It became evident that he had little to no self-love and self-compassion. In fact, what manifested as one of his goals was that he wanted to be able to walk into his local sports club or into a bar with his eyes looking forward not downwards, and literally be able to have eye contact with people, smile and say, 'Hi, can I buy you a drink?' That was it, that was his goal, or one of them.

We worked hard together meeting every week. Seeing that we were making notable progress, I asked him if he would be interested in working on an affirmation. There are many definitions of affirmation, one very simple; 'a statement that something is true'. That's it, you must believe it to be true or it will never contribute to any growth. He came back with, 'I want to feel free to be me'. This was very interesting as what he was referring to was actually his goal for life. Just to like, and eventually love, who he was.

Another issue was that this affirmation was in the future tense and affirmations need to be in the present tense. It's no good reminding yourself of what you're going to be as, in a way, you are repeating what you are presently not! You have to start believing right away. It would have been more powerful to say, 'I'm now free to be me'. We had a lot more work to do.

So, what did we do?

We got stuck into a coaching journey of total commitment plus the other five pillars of the way. This has now become cemented into my coaching system. We built an impregnable fortress (belief structure) over time and then relentlessly unpacked some areas of need by setting some clear and inspirational goals. Basically, we stripped everything back to find honesty and clarity.

We worked hard on targeting his self-belief system and we made sure he started the day with the poem 'The Man in the Glass' as a routine. He decided to print the poem and mount it on the wall. You should be familiar with this poem by now, too. He did the same with his values, printed them off and placed them where he would see them the most, at home and at work.

When the time was right we revisited another affirmation that he would either mentally acknowledge or speak out loud every time he looked in the mirror. In the morning brushing his teeth, or when catching a glimpse of himself in a shop window or the rear-view mirror in his car.

The affirmation he came up with was 'I HAVE THE POWER'. We had worked so hard together that he reached a point whereby he truly felt that he had the power to achieve anything he put his mind to. By then we'd flipped his perception of life into seeing that it was actually full of opportunity, it was abundant and, yes, at times, very challenging but it no longer consisted of bad luck and failure.

From that moment, I finished all my recap notes, emails and text messages to him with 'remember, I HAVE THE POWER', making sure every communication reaffirmed this belief.

It was phrased in the present tense, and it started to become reality for him. He really started to understand that he 'had the power' to transcend, he 'had the power' to put his mind to anything. He 'had the power' to change his life. Anything was achievable.

So, what happened next?...

Soon after, he nailed his short-term goal of making eye contact with people and became much more socially capable.

On the 31st July, 2019 around 7.00 pm in the evening, just before our coaching session, my client was pacing around in another part of the hotel lounge where we had our sessions together, deliberating texting a lady to ask her out. He told me a week later he had the text typed out, all he had to do was press send! He felt he was in a place, for the first time in years, whereby he'd discovered the inner confidence and self-belief to send a text to this woman he could not stop thinking about.

Sweating profusely and trying to recapture my notes and what he had learned about himself, relating back to his values, his fortress and the anti-procrastination tools we covered, he pressed 'send'!

We got straight into the coaching session. My client never mentioned what he had just done. The session ended and he glanced at his phone. There was a message, it was from the woman he had sent the text to. It read: *'I have been waiting two years to receive this!'* It was sent two minutes after his!

How wonderful! Just nine weeks after our first session together my client had found the mental strength and inner resources to make such a bold move. As I write this book, this gentleman is still my client, and I can share with you that he and his partner are deeply in love, have moved out of their respective houses, bought a house together and are planning a family.

He is now making the most of this amazing opportunity to spend the rest of his life with this person, which nine weeks before was just wishful thinking, it was literally a pipe dream.

In addition, my client has fulfilled another ambition, to work for himself and rid himself of the 'bully boss'.

This is what true and meaningful self-belief and self-value can deliver. I feel truly honoured to be a part of that magnificent story. He certainly had the power! There's a movie in there somewhere!

The forthcoming green belt syllabus offers you more response tools that will allow you to combat, control and defeat the stress that comes at us both extrinsically (the outside world) and intrinsically (from our own thinking, our inner world). It's designed to help you understand what actually occurs in our bodies, from the miraculous inborn systems we have, to the damage we can do to ourselves from our own thinking. In the past, I have described my own negative thinking as a form of self-harming.

So, the tools are corrective actions but you will see along the way that the more you train the less likely it is you will need them. You'll actually grow and establish your own preventative filters to stop stress from reaching the hotspots in the first place.

Karate is a wonderful example of something that can reduce stress. Why? Obviously, it's well known that exercise does this with lots of positive neurochemistry being produced during the exercise routine, but more importantly it allows you to focus your mind on something other than your stress. This is why I felt so refreshed and why I was buzzing every time I left the dojo.

So why can't we devise some tools to help us deal with stress in real time by tweaking the way we process what we are experiencing? The Health and Safety Executive (HSE) reports in a Labour Force Survey that, in 2019/20 17.9 million days were lost due to work-related stress, depression or anxiety. Staggering figures I'm sure you would agree.

Those stress or threat response hormones, epinephrine and cortisol, are magnificent for short bursts. But too much of them in your system too often can have a negative effect and produce chronic symptoms such as blood sugar imbalance, higher blood pressure, increase in weight and lowered immunity. These reactions could potentially trigger even more serious consequences relating to heart problems, high cholesterol and strokes. Lower level consequences are a decrease in cognition, perception, collaboration and creativity. When stressed it becomes incredibly challenging to solve problems and work with other people.

I must also mention that there is such a thing as good stress. We need some degree of stress to get us out of bed in the morning. Psychologists refer to it as 'eustress'. This is when we feel excited and start to experience a similar response to bad stress, such as an increase in heart rate. We have a surge in hormonal activity and yet there is no threat at all. Why is this? The globally recognised coach, author and speaker Tony Robins tells an amazing story in his audio book *Unleash the Power Within* about two of his famous clients – singer-songwriter Carly Simon and the legendary Bruce Springsteen. Tony was interested to learn how they prepared and what they both experienced before going on stage to perform in front of thousands of people.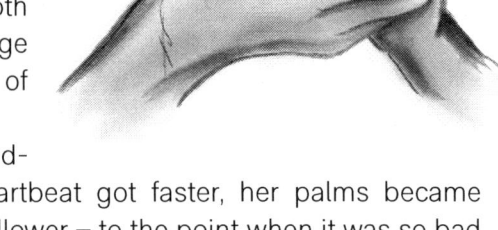

Carly Simon described the lead-up to a performance as; her heartbeat got faster, her palms became sweaty, her breathing became shallower – to the point when it was so bad she had a panic attack and sometimes couldn't go on stage.

Bruce Springsteen described his lead-up as; his heartbeat got faster, his palms became sweaty, his breathing became shallower – to the point when he felt he had reached a peak physical state of alertness and he was ready and primed to perform.

Similar responses in physiology but opposite mindsets. Absolutely incredible!

It's OK to get nervous, it's your body's way of preparing for something you might deem as challenging. Most of us get nervous when experiencing a new opportunity – these are feelings to embrace and not dispel.

I could never understand why, when playing cricket, I always got nervous before I went into bat. Even if I had scored a 100 in the previous game, I was well prepared and even if I was playing against the lowest side in the league with a poor bowling attack – I still became nervous. I would get butterflies in my stomach, a rise in my breathing and sweaty palms. I now know it was my mind and body preparing itself, in the same way Bruce

Springsteen experienced, before performing. I wish I had understood this then as I used to give myself a hard time for feeling that way. I thought I was suffering from a lack of confidence. That wasn't the case – it was just another natural miracle going on inside me. However, nervousness, like many things, can persist and grow into anxiety or phobia. We will cover ways to combat this during our green belt syllabus.

It is for you to absorb, digest, practise and deliver on the road to self-mastery and living a black belt life. But it all starts and finishes with the power of the mind. As we move closer to the black belt, we will discover the technique for finding the 'sweet spot' of performance when we need it most. For this magic to occur I will help you to manage, regulate and support these body and mind miracles to your advantage giving you the edge over and above the rest.

So, we have learnt that we all have an inborn emergency service that we don't even have to make a call to or connect with. It's instinctive and instantaneous. As stated, it has been referred to as 'fight or flight' or your survival system. A miracle of nature, it just deals with situations in a split second and can produce extraordinary results.

We now also realise we can activate this emergency service by our thinking and convert this incredible innate life-saving capability into something that can become quite harmful if our thinking spirals out of control, causing us anxiety, panic and other forms of stress that can result in long-lasting and devastating illness.

Just by understanding what goes on inside of you, even in a small way, will help you with immediate effect as you begin to recognise certain stress-related signals. You'll identify what's happening further in advance or take a look inside yourself and acknowledge what's occurring.

It's a bit like writing a 'to do list' – it immediately makes you more effective. Understanding yourself from the inside out does exactly the same.

YELLOW BELT GRADING WARM-UP:

This syllabus was dedicated to building on your platform of learning and creativity, taking the skill of self-awareness into the brain, body and mind which, in turn, helps you to identify, respond, manage and control both outside and inside world stressors, a gigantic step to living a black belt life.

We covered the innate miracle of our survival system designed to take care of us when faced with danger and the inconceivable physiology and speed of reaction behind the fight or flight response to a serious threat.

It was made clear that threats, danger and stress can also be an inside job, created by our own imagination, our own thinking. We can literally create situations in our minds or relive past traumatic experiences, designing virtual events that set off our survival system and the more we do it the greater potential for long-term chronic disorders.

We looked at the three fears and how they are mindset driven, developed over years of growing up and how we can distort our thinking to a storyline only limited to the boundary of the fantasy.

The power of the mind is almost beyond words. Yes, there is a dark side but there is also light. Brilliant, glistening light, a positively transformational life-changing light that is at the heart of success and fulfilment. We looked at the placebo as a measure of what the mind can help achieve in the form of purified, totally devoted belief.

We touched on the influence that the skill of holding attention can produce and the by-products from this and the myth of multitasking also.

We covered the destructive nature of distraction and how we can become much more effective with a minimal understanding of how our brains work.

This syllabus provided you with the necessary training to allow you to look further, deeper, longer inside of yourself to help you to manage, regulate, control and respond to situations that challenge you from the outside world or sometimes manifest psychologically from the inside world and as a yellow belt going for green belt, we cover something that can, in itself, change your life forever.

Good luck with your yellow belt grading.

YELLOW BELT GRADING

1. Recap your learning from your book of life by checking into your orange and red belt key points including reading 'The Man in the Glass' again to create the right mental activity and attitude.
2. Reflect, explore and identify your fight and flight experiences intrinsically and extrinsically. Is there any learning to be gained from this? Can you now identify with the physiology that occurred?
3. Are you aware of past cognitive distortions you have experienced and, moving forward, what tools could you deploy to help?
4. Work on your attention skills, your concentration levels, being able to focus and avoid distraction. How can you develop this area of your life? What results might you see?
5. Look at what distracts you. What's getting in the way of your performance and untapped potential and how can you reshape your work life to become more effective?
6. Check in to see how mentally exhausted you become some days. Then out your schedule and how many plates you were spinning.
7. List six key takeaways from this syllabus.

Congratulations!
You are now a yellow belt.

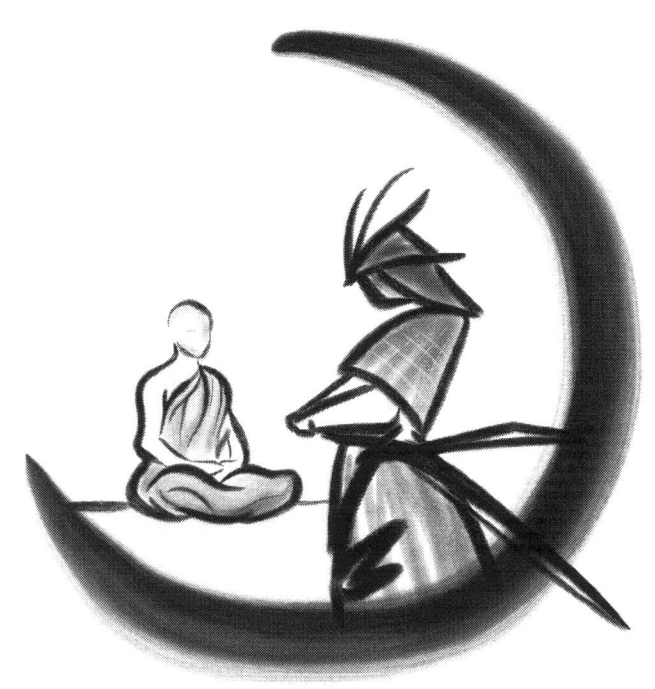

CHAPTER 5
GREEN BELT
A Mind Less Full

'Live the actual moment. Only this actual moment is life'. ~ THICH NHAT HANN

You now have reached a deeper understanding of the journey; the way.

So far, you have developed your mental and spiritual core strength by building a strong and powerful belief structure, including your value system, which will dictate your behaviour and guide you through life like an inbuilt radar and navigation system. You have created a natural go-to healing and protection system in the form of gratefulness and a willingness to help others, as well as being honest and open about your fears and self-limitations and facing them as part of the fortress model.

You have unpacked some of your key strengths, successes and accomplishments, designed and painted exciting life-changing pictures of what your future looks like in the form of a unique and transformational goal-setting process. You have also increased your self-esteem, inner belief and confidence levels, which should all be rapidly rising, confirming you are on the way to transcending to something very special.

In addition to all this, you have looked inside the mind and brain to discover the complex but incredible powers of each entity. This entire book is based around developing a positive attitude and the realisation that we can all control our thoughts and responses to create better outcomes.

The last chapter looked at situations out of our control that ignite our rapid response survival system. Nevertheless, the same system can become permanently in play through our own catastrophic thinking causing us both mental and physical harm. Through the yellow belt syllabus, we achieved a better understanding of the destructive nature of stress on the body, mind and soul. We've learned about the power of the mind and how, if used effectively, it can provide all the necessary inner tools and external radars to spot incoming threats and deal with them effectively, preventing them from developing into something much worse with potentially devastating consequences. One way of looking at this is by having two minds; the thinking mind and the observer, the watcher. This means stepping outside of your own experience and looking in at what's occurring. I cannot express how helpful this is. Alone, this skill is transformational.

THE MONK AND THE SAMURAI

Stress is brought into our lives by the way we process and respond to outer world events but also the inner world cognitive journeys we take. I'm now going to explain ways to construct additional layers of personal protection to greater strengthen your inner skills and self-confidence that simply alters your interpretation and response to such events. This will help you to live your life by design. It's your life – you should be the person who chooses how it plays out.

In martial arts, to reach high performance levels, you need to be calm and relaxed, have a laser-like focus and a sixth sense awareness, while in total control. This is something you master through the transition of colours from white to black and beyond. This is precisely what we are going to explore in this green belt syllabus. These skills, this mindset, the specific art of self-awareness is what separates the best from the rest, not just in the dojo but in everyday life.

You can now see how building a personal belief structure raises inner confidence and self-esteem. It fires up self-belief to levels never previously experienced and helps you find greater clarity. Add to it a little more understanding as to your physiology and the fundamental need to manage and regulate emotions and stresses, we can achieve more clarity about what your life design looks like. I liken these breakthroughs, insights, tools and learning to a sort of spiritual Personal Protective Equipment (PPE) that keep you safe from the winds of life that blow on us every day.

I spent many years working with highly sophisticated personal protection systems that were designed using the latest blast and fire-resistant fabric technology, mostly Kevlar. Many layers of material made from tightly woven fibres provide protection against the force of a blast by spreading the impact over a large surface area.

This multi-layered, blast-proof suit feels like the perfect analogy to what I want to provide you with; your own mind, body and soul personal protection system to combat the many inner and outer world battles we face. The tools from this syllabus and others in this book, when woven together, like the fibres described, deliver amazing resistance to the outside forces that emerge as stress, anxiety, regret, guilt, negativity and worse. We will, therefore, now focus on one of the most remarkable of life's gemstones in the form of ancient Buddhist wisdom – mindfulness.

I personally discovered mindfulness many years ago from one of the two 'angels' I have met in my life so far, long before it became as popular as it is now. In recent years it's been recognised as a way to manage mental health and reduce stress. It's now taught in schools, hospitals, even prisons and the military. Today, mindfulness has become a growing trend in business as reduced stress levels equate to happier people, which results in greater productivity and so on. And, I am delighted to inform you, it works.

Before we begin, I feel it fitting to afford you yet more good news…you don't have to go anywhere to find mindfulness, you already have it, locked away, as does every single human being on the planet. You were born with it. Now let's learn how to embrace it!

In this grade we are going to expand on *Mokuso,* the silent mind, the meditative beginning and end to a karate training session that I referred to in the white belt syllabus. I said how wonderful it would be to start and end every day the same way, with *Mokuso.* Focus in the morning and reflection at night. But how about taking it a step further, altering the bit between the beginning and the end to live a life of mindfulness.

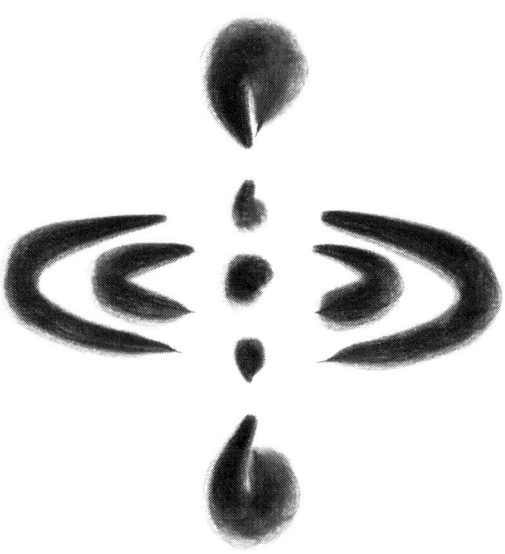

WHAT IS MINDFULNESS?

Let me start by telling you what I feel it's not. It's not purely sitting cross-legged in a candlelit room doing breathing exercises, wiping your mind of all its clutter and noise; although this example of meditation offers immense value to your overall well-being, and meditation and yoga are still at the heart of modern mindfulness.

I view meditation as a practice, hugely fulfilling but a practice nonetheless. It's intended to create a heightened state of awareness, a calmness and peace using the discipline of concentration and focussing on the breath. This keeps you in the present moment and helps you take control of your state of mind. You can become extremely competent at this and it will most definitely provide you with many wellness-related benefits. As a child, I can remember my mum saying to me 'take some deep breaths' if I was nervous about something. I'm sure we have all been told that at least once in our lives. Mum didn't appreciate that what she was offering was a practice dating back thousands of years, a meditation which is a countermeasure for anxiety and suffering. I still see it as a drill and, just like *Mokuso*, it can become part of your daily rituals and develop into mindfulness and a mindful way of living.

I believe that mindfulness is a wisdom – 'a way'. It's an awareness, an attitude, an incredible way of living and, I assure you all, a pathway to happiness.

The word mindfulness is a translation of 'sati', a word from the Pali language of ancient India, in which many original Buddhist texts were written. Roughly translated, it means 'awareness, attention and remembering'. The remembering part of the trinity is remembering to be aware and remembering to pay attention.

Mindfulness, on its own, has countless benefits and can offer a major shift in your life if you practise it, but when you incorporate mindfulness into living a black belt life, then the transition leads to something quite remarkable. We have reached the stage of the way where an awakening can occur, transforming your life.

Mindfulness has evolved from its Buddhist roots dating back over 2500 years. Buddha actually means 'the enlightened one' or 'the awakened one'. One of his students asked the Buddha, 'Are you God?'

'No,' replied the Buddha.

'Then are you a healer?'

'No,' replied the Buddha.

'Then are you a teacher?'

'No, I am not a teacher.'

'Then what are you?' asked the student.

'I am awake,' said the Buddha.

Awake or awareness is what mindfulness represents.

Awareness can be broken down into many elements. Mindfulness tunes in to a particular type of self-awareness that maintains a moment-by-moment consciousness or understanding of our feelings and the surrounding environment. The secret is that mindfulness plays out life, in real time, which has also been described as 'the now', seeing things as they really are in that moment.

So many of us, me included, spend our lives either stuck in our past or focussing on the future, or both, and forget to centre on the here and now. These mindsets generally produce feelings of regret, guilt and self-reproach when we journey back to our past. Or anxiety, uncertainty, pressure and stress when our thinking takes us to the future.

John Kabat-Zin, an American professor of medicine referred to as the 'godfather of modern mindfulness', defines mindfulness as, *'the awareness that arises from paying attention, on purpose, in the present moment and non-judgementally'.*

Holding on to, or carrying resentment and grudges from past events, eventually takes its toll and becomes a weight on our shoulders. I know I've done it myself. When I reflect on the years I chose to hold on to this mentality towards various events that occurred in my life I realise what resulted from that thinking was pure negative energy. I couldn't change what occurred yet I made the decision, time and time again, to revisit it in my head. It can manifest anger or regret, bitterness, even jealousy. I've heard it said that life is short but we don't know how short. Yet we allow our mind to infringe on our precious time and transport us to these toxic places. We all have stories to tell relating to this.

Letting go can be such a liberating

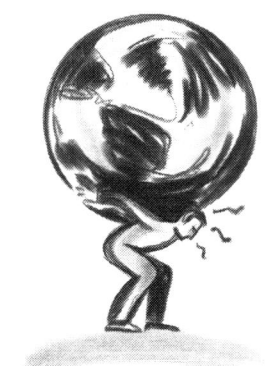

experience. Surrender and acceptance is another way of putting it. Let me explain, as this is extremely important. Surrender does not mean giving up. Surrender in this context is an amazing strength, not a weakness. It takes courage to let go, it's an awesome tool of life.

There is a wonderful Zen parable that puts it all in perspective.

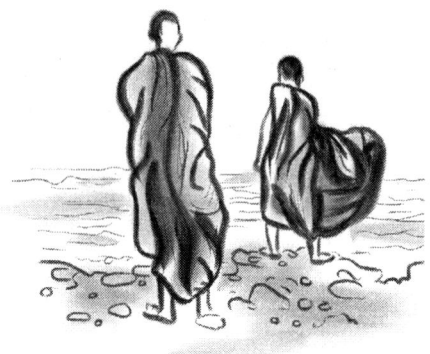

A senior monk and a junior monk were travelling together. At one point, they came to a river with a strong current. As the monks were preparing to cross the river, they saw a beautiful, young woman, alone, also attempting to cross. The young woman asked if they could help her cross to the other side as the current was too strong for her.

The two monks glanced at one another because they had taken vows not to touch a woman. Then, without a word, the older monk picked up the woman, carried her across the river, placed her gently on the other side, and carried on his journey.

The younger monk couldn't believe what had just happened, he was speechless, appalled at what he had just witnessed. An hour passed without a word between them.

Two more hours passed, then three, finally the younger monk could contain himself no longer, and blurted out, 'As monks, we are not permitted to touch a woman, how could you then carry that woman on your shoulders?'

The older monk replied, 'Brother, I set her down hours ago by the side of the river, why are you still carrying her?'

An amazing message reminding us not to dwell on the past and hang on to bad stuff that's happened in the form of resentment or guilt. What good does it do? The fact is that we are only hurting ourselves and dwelling in the past takes away from the present.

We all get hurt on occasion, for sure, we are only human and it's natural we feel this way at times. We all have feelings. But remember our thinking is a choice. The more we focus on the grudge, resentment, or guilt the heavier it becomes and will just weigh us down. Therefore, we can choose to put it down by the side of the river and move on and focus on the present. This is really where true life exists, in the present moment.

Why live in the past as we cannot change it? It's impossible to predict and exist in the future, so why live life worrying about what might or might not happen? That leaves only this present and precious moment that we should make the most of; don't waste your life stuck in the past, make the most of it right now.

It sounds simple enough, but it's not. Like everything we do, to get good at it we need to practise, learn and develop; but we have to start somewhere and that's at the beginning, the now, right now.

In karate we are constantly learning and developing new physical skills, one after the other, and then relentlessly repeating them, honing them, aiming for mastery. We can also apply this to mindfulness. As I sit here writing with the sun streaming through the window, listening to birds singing in the trees, I am in the moment, the here and now, and it's a truly beautiful feeling.

Before we go into more detail about mindfulness and its incredible benefits, it's only fair that I share with you my own story of discovery and the life-changing breakthrough it gave me, during a dark period of my life. I experienced some life challenges that, to many, would not be deemed as significantly damaging but I got stuck in a story of negativity and became downbeat and dispirited, eventually replacing my self-confidence with self-pity,

The way I am going to convey this to you is a little different to the norm. Let me explain…

As a coach who includes mindfulness as part of my coaching model, I was invited to speak at the most amazing venue in London. Built in 1928, this oak-panelled Grade I listed building seats around 170 people plus standing room in the galleries, allowing for well over 200 people at any one event.

The venue hosts regular weekly lectures as a continuing professional development programme. Knowing I was booked to speak about mindfulness, I asked if I could attend the event arranged for the week before to get a feel for how the proceedings unfold. This was sanctioned so I arrived in good time for the event. I got my security pass and was then directed to the room. I was the first one there. It was simply magnificent. I looked around and up at the galleries. What a building, just incredible. I looked at the stage and the lectern placed on it and thought: *It will be me standing there this time next week.*

People started to arrive, and I took my seat. Once the speaker was ready to start, I looked around to see that the downstairs seating was roughly half full and the galleries almost empty apart from one or two people. *That's OK, I thought, not too intimidating,* and gauged the attendance to be the normal turnout.

I couldn't have been more wrong.

The following week I turned up, early as usual, and again I was the first there. I was sharing the talk with a coaching colleague of mine. We had planned a lecture about the benefits of mindfulness under the auspices of mental health strategies for the workplace.

I did another look around and sucked in the positive energy I was getting from being alone in the venue.

People started to arrive – the hosts, the secretary, the chairperson and then the audience. One by one, then a few more. I took my position on the far left at the top table on the stage as I was first up after the introductions.

People were still entering, then more and more. It was getting close to the start time. The seating area downstairs was now full, with more people still arriving! By now there was standing room only at the sides of the room. My eyes were fixed in front of me due to the amount of people present. I had forgotten about the galleries! I looked up and saw they were also crammed with people. There was no space left for anyone. The place was absolutely packed to the rafters. I was later advised this was a turnout that hadn't been seen for a long time.

There followed silence, complete quietness, with no rustling nor movement. The announcements started with introductions then health and safety procedures and so on. Next up it was me! The chairperson introduced me.

Here is my talk, it's almost verbatim as I delivered it...

Ladies and gentlemen,
I would like to share with you a story about someone who is very close to me. His name is Fred. I have called the story...

THE AMAZING FRED

Fred had a modest, humble but happy upbringing and education. He started work in a factory, aged seventeen, as a trainee electronics engineer. After working there for a while, he looked up into the offices and saw people dressed in smart jackets, shirts and ties and thought: That's what I want to do. That's what I want to wear to go to work!

Not long after, Fred had a great office job wearing a smart jacket, shirt and tie.

More time passed and Fred met people who had the luxury of company cars as part of their work package. Fred thought it would be just fantastic to have a company car! I want a job with a company car, he thought.

Fred soon had a job with his own company car!

So, Fred was now wearing a suit, shirt and tie to work and driving a company car! Wow!

Fred was a good sportsman. He was school football captain and a successful cricket club captain but then he wanted to test his leadership skills off the sports field in the business arena. Soon an opportunity came along which Fred took and he fast-tracked his way to the top of an organisation, as high up as he could get, reporting to the owners.

Years passed by and Fred had another ambition to become a business owner, he achieved this too and with his business partner they enjoyed great success.

Alongside Fred's shining career he continued to enjoy his success in sport. He was a good footballer earning trials for professional clubs. He was an even better cricketer. He joined a club; broke many records and he became one of most successful players and captains in his club's 135-year history.

Fred was in awe of martial artists and in his forties he took up karate.

Not happy with just participating, Fred wanted to become a black belt.

Fred trained and trained and became a black belt. Then he trained even more to get his instructor's licence and became a karate instructor.

Fred got the girl! In the 1980s, Fred met a beautiful girl, got married in the Seychelles and they had a beautiful daughter.

Ambitious Fred now had his sights on the big house in the country. He got it. Then he wanted a bigger house with a swimming pool. He got that, too. Next was the super car and the big 4x4 on the driveway. And then the ultimate...the place in the sun. He also got all those things.

So, ladies and gentlemen, in the goldfish bowl of life, everyone looking into Fred's life thought: Wow, Fred has it all. He had the business, the money, the houses, the cars, beautiful family – and the black belt!

FRED HAD IT ALL!

Or did he?

Fred suffered with two severe bouts of mental illness.

The first time was when he was pushing his way to the top of an organisation. One day Fred hit a mental wall. He had nothing left, total fatigue, mental burnout. Having no energy left, Fred was literally spent.

Fred wouldn't go to the doctor as he was in fear of being signed off work. And that to Fred was total failure – failure in terms of his ego and, so he thought, in the eyes of the people he was working for.

Miraculously, Fred got through this bout of illness on his own, only to suffer again years later. But this time it was worse, far worse. This time it manifested itself in the form of severe depression.

Fred described this like slipping down a black hole of life. And the black hole was full of self-pity, insecurity, jealousy, anger, negativity and bad luck.

Fred used all his core values, including resilience and resolve, and also his competitiveness to reach out to find something to grab hold of to pull himself out of this hole. But he couldn't find anything to grab on to and he began to slip further and further downwards.

He started to suffer with a type of social phobia whereby he would cross the road and hide to avoid people he knew.

Ladies and gentlemen, Fred was in a bad way!

Until one day, on a train to London, he met a mindfulness teacher. He was sitting directly opposite him. He had been briefly introduced to him a few weeks before. The mindfulness teacher said, 'Hi, how are you?'

Awkwardly, Fred replied, 'Well, a bit stressed, you know how it is, normal stuff.'

The mindfulness teacher looked at Fred and said, 'Fred, I feel your pain, I really do. Do me a favour, just hold your hands out in front of you and close your eyes, just for thirty seconds. And bring your attention to your fingertips. If your mind or your attention wanders just gently bring it back to your fingertips. They might start to tingle but that's OK.'

Fred did exactly this. After thirty seconds the teacher said, 'OK, open your eyes and tell me how you feel.'

Fred opened his eyes and looked around and said, 'I feel great.'

The mindfulness teacher said, 'For thirty seconds, I took you away from your past, your regrets and frustrations. I brought you back from the future we seem to spend our lives trying to burst into. Worrying about what may or may not happen in our lives and the anxiety and emotions attached to it. Fred, for thirty seconds you were just in the here and now. For those seconds you experienced mindfulness.'

Fred had an instant epiphany. He realised he was feeling the sum total of his thoughts, his thinking, it was like he had been mentally self-harming.

From that moment Fred continued to study and practise mindfulness. Those thirty seconds changed Fred's life forever. The world that surrounds Fred is still the same, but he looks at it through different lenses. Now he looks at the same world of self-pity, insecurity and bad luck as a world of opportunity, prosperity and wonder, along with compassion and empathy, and all without judgement.

I then asked the audience: 'What are the takeaways from Fred's story?' I went on to explain:

1. Never ever take anyone's mental health for granted.
2. To all the leaders and bosses out there. It's so important to create a safe and secure environment at work, a structure and pathway to allow people the opportunity to discuss and talk about their mental health challenges at work.
3. To all the Freds and Fredas out there. There is a way out, there is light at the end of the tunnel and Fred is living proof of this.

Ladies and gentlemen, before I hand you back, I would like to share one last thing with you. Some of you might have guessed already that…

Fred is actually me!

It feels quite strange sharing this story for the first time with so many people I have never met, when I couldn't share it with the people I was closest to when I was suffering.

If I knew then what I know now, obviously life would have been different. But I needed to go on that journey to be in a position to help others take on

and defeat their mental challenges as well as reach and fulfil their goals and dreams. Thank you.

I was met with an unexpected, lengthy and moving round of applause. I believed the protocol was to only clap at the end of the entire event, so it was very touching indeed.

When we had finished, I had a queue of people lining up to speak to me. It was quite surreal, but I had some quality time to reflect on this awe-inspiring experience on my train journey home.

I was soon invited back to do another event, then another...

On reflection, I think I suffered with four episodes of depression as an adult, not two, all at different degrees of severity and at different times of my life. However, I was living proof of the power of mindfulness to all those people, professionals from different levels and walks of life. I guess they needed to hear that it's OK not to be OK sometimes. And that help is out there and, more importantly, help is in there too, already tucked away within us.

So, this was my way of explaining my introduction to mindfulness to an audience on that day and now it includes you, my kind readers, who are on the special journey of the way.

I have also introduced you to one of my angels whom I met on the train. We have all met people who have helped us, that were inspirational, achievers, really cool people, someone to look up to. Family, teachers, friends, work colleagues, but this chance meeting on a train changed my life from that moment.

My personal study and exploration of mindfulness, and ensuing learning since then has taught me so much. The results have been transformational and, to this day, I'm still learning and improving. I have woven mindfulness into my daily life, from the inside out and outside in, and my life is the better for it. This proves, once again, what the masterful Jim Rohn said, that the greatest gift you can give anybody is your own personal development. I can honestly say that adopting a more mindful approach to life, benefits all the people you encounter, every single person, every single day.

I can best describe mindfulness as a magnificent tool, the best tool in the kitbag to help alleviate suffering and guide you to a safe and peaceful place. This underpins how it emanated from Buddhism, almost as a system or antidote to combat both physical and psychological suffering, which, as we know, is often self-inflicted.

The engaging spiritual leader Sadhguru says we experience pain to preserve ourselves as part of our survival system. Suffering, however, is something that happens in your mind. Ironically, two of our greatest natural gifts are what causes our suffering in the first place; a vivid memory and a fantastic imagination. We can still suffer from events that occurred years ago but also from what we believe the future holds. Isn't that so true? Fred can vouch for this.

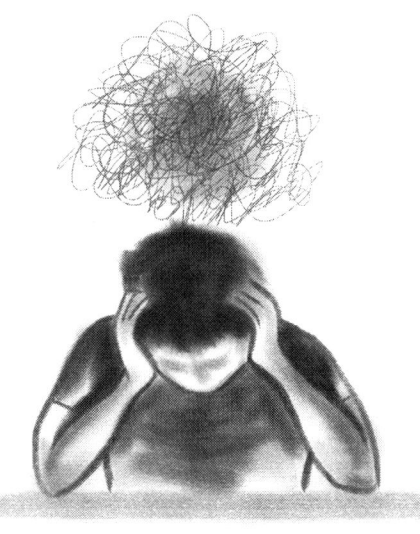

We will find out later that mindfulness can actually change your brain. Some people believe mindfulness is the opposite to mindlessness, of which we have all experienced on more than one occasion. Have you ever driven the same route home for years and then missed a turning because your mind is elsewhere? This is mindlessness.

In our crazy, frantic worlds of processing endless streams of information, no wonder we suffer at times with information overload. We are on a journey, constantly reacting and responding to events, always learning and dealing with ever-changing challenges, constantly moving on to the next task at hand, and the next. Ask yourselves this – are you ever really paying attention to what you're doing? No, of course you're not.

On top of this we are bombarded with daily brainwashing through social media, TV, radio, magazines, and other mediums as to what we should look like, wear, drive, eat, drink, how we should behave, parent and so on. It's no wonder our minds become overwhelmed, our minds are so full of noise – cluttered, jammed and frazzled. Our modern headspace has been likened to a box of flies or bees with so many thoughts buzzing around in our heads to the point where you cannot think straight. A Buddhist term is 'monkey mind', meaning unsettled and restless with the mind jumping from thought to thought like a monkey from tree to tree. I know there will be many of you nodding as you read this, thinking, *that's me!*

Then there's our need to compare ourselves with others. Comparison is the shortcut to misery, by the way. We see people thinner, fitter, wealthier, smarter, more successful, happier people than us, and so on. The aforementioned simply blocks the route to happiness and can develop into stress and exhaustion, which leads to that downward spiral to anxiety and depression. These are perfect examples of work-life experiences that put us into that fight or flight mode as described in the yellow belt syllabus. We continue to flood ourselves with our primeval life-saving neurochemistry, which in constant supply does much more harm than good.

Now I'm going to throw in something else. Our negativity bias which I alluded to earlier on our journey, another evolutionary hand-me-down. I'm afraid this is still with us from the early days of our caveman existence whereby we constantly scanned for threats due to a life-or-death existence. This is why negative events imprint more rapidly and stay longer than positive ones. They are much more powerful.

I like the example of the boss that sits down with you and delivers your annual review. He has six points. The first five are excellent but the last is negative relating to an area that you need to develop. What do you take home with you? The five good points or the one negative point. I'll let you answer that as I already know the answer.

Another example, Danny Kahneman, who won the 2002 Nobel Prize designed a study whereby people imagined either winning or losing $50. Even though the amount was the same the emotional reaction was considerably greater for those imagining what it would be like to lose the money. The negativity of losing something was far greater than the positivity of gaining something. This is our negative bias in action.

Furthermore, we are always trying to get rid of a moment to get to another better moment. We are trying to get through one part of our life to get to another. Get to work to get home to see the kids. Get the kids to bed to watch a movie. Get the gym out of the way so I can enjoy my dinner. Get dinner over so I can work… Can you see where I'm going? Always looking to get into the future but never actually getting there as it's impossible.

Another example, imagine you've never set foot in a dojo, and you arrive for your first ever karate lesson…

If I was to say to you as my student, 'OK, these are the correct stances, hand and elbow positions, knees bent and flexed at all times, weight distribution must be around 70% on the back leg for a back stance, focus on your core and centre of gravity, keep a straight back and good posture at all times.' I then demonstrate the correct movement forward, to the side and backwards and so on. If I then said to you, 'Away you go let's see what you can do.' I think you might spontaneously combust in front of my eyes! You'd probably have a mental meltdown and, most likely, never turn up again.

Information overload results in the conscious, decision-making part of the brain, the PFC we looked at in the yellow belt syllabus, shutting down. This is the sort of thing that we are subliminally being faced with every day of our lives. It's no wonder we feel tired, fatigued, worn out, burnt out, stuck in our narrative and operating on pure autopilot. It's no surprise we struggle to feel happy, content, creative and forward-thinking, or be a positive influence, motivational and inspirational to others. All in all, each and every one of us is in desperate need of a little quietness, space and peace, reflection and inner tranquillity. At times, life can literally drain your brain.

I am thrilled to be able to deliver some wonderful news in this chapter. Pay attention…allowing mindfulness into your life can help dilute, and eventually remove, these daily, draining, brain-sapping responses to your existence. It doesn't have to be like this. Mindfulness helps us to manage, regulate and control our lives. The result is that it provides an area of peace, just for you, and you can keep it forever. It's yours and is always there for you to visit. It takes us away from ego, and the constant use of 'me' and 'I' in our thoughts and language. It connects us to a world outside of ourselves. It helps us to see things for what they are rather than what we'd like them to be. And it helps us to experience the joy and richness of each moment and acknowledge thoughts and feelings as they manifest themselves.

It helps us with relationships and not to take things so personally. It even helps with our brain circuitry. There is a great deal of scientific support and endorsement for mindfulness being at the pinnacle of psychotherapeutic interventions. And, undoubtedly, it helps us press pause and take a breath before we respond to situations.

All of this and more. Mindfulness helps us to live our life in a richer, more fulfilling and happier way. It's part of the way to a black belt life.

Mindfulness has proven to help with many other things too, such as:

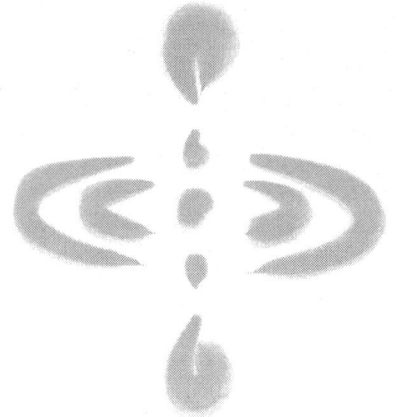

- Reducing stress
- Decreasing anxiety
- Decreasing blood pressure
- Pain management
- Improving sleep
- Depressive symptoms
- General mental health
- Boosting the immune system
- Greater concentration skills
- Feeling of positivity
- Inner peace and love

So, how do we cultivate a more mindful way of living? It is about paying greater attention to what you are doing right now and cultivating the intention to keep doing it. It's simply – 'paying attention with intention'.

Again referencing David Rock's book, *Your Brain at Work*, leading mindfulness researcher John Teasdale, says, '*Mindfulness is a habit, it's a skill that can be learnt, it's accessing something we already have. Mindfulness isn't difficult, what's difficult is remembering to be mindful.*'

This doesn't mean that we cannot plan for the future or set goals. As a coach, part of my model uses a successful goal-creating and setting process along with my studies and practice of mindfulness and neuroscience. I had to wrestle with what I thought to be a contradiction to my philosophy. Mindfulness is about being present, experiencing life moment-by-moment, whereas goal creating involves visualisation, planning and aiming for future triumphs and success. This was my dilemma, so I had to dig deep to search for a little much-needed wisdom.

One day when running this conundrum through my mind for the umpteenth time, I felt a warming smile appearing and a glow of satisfaction flowing throughout my body due to the mini-epiphany I had just experienced. And now it has become part of my goal-creating and setting strategy.

So, my insight was this…

If you remember in the red belt chapter, the goal-setting process needs to be incredibly meticulous in its detail, this is key. It must also meet specific criterion to qualify as a goal. If you adhere to these requirements, together they will deliver the necessary clarity any goal must have for it to work.

Once the process has been scrupulously designed and it's managed by the six pillars of the way, it allows you to experience your life in the present moment. It essentially provides a platform for a more mindful approach that takes care of future pressures and worries. This is because you have what the brain adores; clarity and certainty.

Focussing on the process, not the goal, helps you to embrace a moment-to-moment experience. You will have prepared brilliantly to allow this to happen, knowing that each step takes you closer to the goal. Two amazing quotes from leadership legend John Maxwell and the master of personal development Jim Rohn offer a kind of freedom and realisation to what goal setting brings to life.

John Maxwell says, 'When you have hope in the future, you have the power in the present.' Whereas Jim Rohn said, 'Learn to be happy with what you have while you pursue all that you want.' This quote from Jim is the last few paragraphs in shorthand! It's saying you can be mindful, happy, grateful while being ambitious and go getting. Perfect, just perfect.

Before I share with you what mindfulness actually means to me, how I have adapted to it and how I have been fortunate to have such a successful relationship with it, I want to bring some scientific support to it. Practising mindfulness can change the way certain regions of the brain communicate with each other. Much research and countless studies have been dedicated to the science of mindfulness. Scientist have used MRI scanning to see how the brain changes during the practice of meditation, certain areas appear to shrink or grow in response to regular mindfulness practice. The amygdala, the brain's stress or fear centre has been shown to shrink, whereby the PFC responsible for planning, setting goals, creativity and solving problems can actually become thicker. It's also said that the hippocampus part, responsible for learning and memory, can also become thicker. It can be argued that 'mindfulness is actually changing our minds and our brains for the better'.

I started to see my mindfulness teacher more and more and attended some of his events. I would meet him at his studio in London, or we would walk along many of the capital's famous streets together.

The truth is, I wasn't very good at meditation. At the start of our meetings my teacher would 'clear the space', a custom that I have adapted and sometimes include in my coaching process. It's basically a version of 'emptying your cup'. Parking or removing the noise and interference of life from our minds. We did this by simply sharing recent thoughts and experiences with each other, which helped to centre us. And then he would take me through breathing exercises that became a more intense type of meditation.

In the beginning, I misunderstood the objective and thought that because I couldn't stop my thinking, I was doing something wrong. I believed the aim was to clear my mind totally from all thought. This was almost impossible for a beginner to meditation. So, I started watching my thoughts, which is what I still do today, but in a more controlled manner.

I didn't realise, at the time, that this is one of the amazing traits of mindfulness. It's called metacognition – thinking about your thinking. It's stepping outside of your experience then tuning in, being more acutely aware of what you are experiencing and simply acknowledging your thoughts and feelings, whatever they are, good or bad, positive or negative. That's it, just acknowledging your thoughts as they come and go without judging them. When you learn to do this, it has a dramatic effect on your emotional control and, subsequently, quality of life.

Then there's meta-awareness, being aware of your awareness. We are the only living thing on the planet with the ability to do this. To check in to our thinking and awareness and then make a choice as to how we respond. I have said this before, I know, but we are living miracles. It's a good feeling to appreciate this in its fullness.

I can best describe this process as stepping outside of what you are experiencing, and observing it as a third person, to see what's actually going on. Observing how you are feeling, what you are thinking and doing, again without any judgement. Just noting and acknowledging what's occurring in the moment even if it's a negative thought. Just acknowledge it's a negative thought, accept it, don't hook it in or engage with it, just move on. This response removes the energy from it and stops it from escalating. The great thing is that you can, with practice, turn this into another superpower. It feels so liberating to have this power I guarantee. When you acquire or develop this strength, your self-confidence unknowingly grows with it.

So, this was something I became really skilled at. It took some time and I'm still working at it. However, it has helped to transform my life. I started to benefit from treating my thoughts as just thoughts, knowing they will come and, more importantly, they will go.

As I became more advanced in my learning, I realised that thinking is a choice, which was so helpful with my personal journey. Another great friend and fellow coach once said to me, *'People get stuck in their own story of thinking, if only they realised, they could change it.'* He's absolutely right.

The fact is that although our thoughts can be so damaging as the 'Amazing Fred' alluded to, they are so incredibly powerful and commanding, which we covered in our yellow belt syllabus. To let you into another secret, as part of my mindfulness apprenticeship I started to practise what I call 'tuning in'. I mentally captured a negative thought that just landed and I know could spiral into something bad. I then mimic grabbing the thought, screwing it up into a ball and throwing it away. I only do it when I'm on my own, though. In the car, I would actually wind the window down and throw it out. I shared this with a client once, and he reported back to say that it helped him, too.

I also became quite skilled at noticing my mood and related thinking to a point whereby I would give myself a quiet once-over, a sort of personal audit. The physical action of screwing up and discarding negativity eventually transitioned into a smile of acknowledgement. I'd smile or chuckle and occasionally say out loud something like, 'I know what you're up to' or, 'how the hell did I let you in? Off you go.' I'm sure there is a technical term for this as it's the next level to metacognition. It's not madness, I can assure you. It's no different than before a match, or presentation, or playing a gig when people shout at themselves, giving that needed boost of adrenaline to pump themselves up.

What I was dealing with was my inner critic; the enemy inside who tricks and torments us. Many of us possess a cruel inner voice. Negative self-talk is like an infection that can become chronic, which so many of us have and cannot get rid of. It can come and go, but with some people it stays, shadowing them like a constant cloud. Another way of dealing with this is when that cruel voice is knocking at our door. Are we going to choose to let it in? We are always ready to help someone else who's struggling with an issue or feeling demotivated. We leap to their support, keen to help them with a boost of inspiration. We listen to them intently and are always quick to provide a shoulder to cry on. So why do we not have the inclination to be kinder, more supportive, compassionate and understanding towards ourselves?

One of the key elements of my clients' successes on their unique and personal journeys is, first and foremost, the effort they put into working on themselves. This is not a selfish act, it's critical to personal growth and transformation. The more time you invest in yourself through mindfulness, personal development and self-discovery, the happier you will become and others around you will benefit too – it's life's positive ripple effect. You will learn so much and reach high levels of fulfilment. Remember one of my favourite quotes from Socrates? 'The unexamined life is not worth living'. Do not stop working on yourself and you will find everything else gets taken care of.

This is what I did to wage a war with my negative thinking...

I started to take control of the inner voice, which was either giving me a hard time, bringing negativity into my mindset by taking me back to the past or making me anxious about the future. Although I started to understand what was going on I still needed a better intervention; another weapon for my arsenal. At first, you never know when the enemy is going to arrive. When you become more advanced, you can spot the enemy from miles away. It's like you have someone on lookout.

Another favourite metaphor to introduce a mindful approach to our thinking is to treat our minds as a beautiful blue sky. The clouds that appear are just thoughts that come and go and that also includes the dark clouds, that negative, destructive, cruel thought. Like the white clouds the dark ones will also pass. Just acknowledge them as thoughts, don't hook into them and wave them past to disappear in the distance leaving that amazing blue sky in their wake.

Being a life and performance coach, I thought it would be a good idea to create an inner coach to combat the inner critic: one v one – the good fighting the bad. The inner coach eventually became my inner samurai and a worthy addition to my fortress. The solitary job of the samurai is to destroy negativity, by flipping it into a positive. So, by finding a positive somewhere in the passage of thought or even checking-in to my belief structure to the chamber where my values, strengths and gratefulness are harnessed, ready to be unleashed, I learned to suppress the negative and remain focussed on the positive. Along with mindfulness, my inner samurai was also armed with some scientifically proven mental tools such as cognitive reappraisal and the positive labelling of emotions.

There are various ways to reappraise a difficult situation and one is altering perspective or changing the direction of thought before it perpetuates into something bad. It's just processing the situation differently. You can become expert at this if you practise. Some people tend to routinely catastrophise situations. An example of this is being stuck in traffic and late for an appointment and construing it as a disaster. Or the football team we support loses an important game. We can be immensely passionate, loyal and committed but if this is the language we are pinning to a late appointment or a game of football then we are setting a dangerous psychological president.

One definition of disaster is 'a sudden accident or a natural catastrophe that causes great damage or loss of life'. Again, it's about perspective, making the choice about which pathway of thought you will take. It's mindset dependent so if we believe something is a disaster, then that's exactly what it will become to you, resulting in the manifestation of the emotions akin to a disaster. The alternative is searching and locating a different spin on the situation.

Another is normalising. I use this technique a great deal when coaching. It's basically acknowledging experiences that lead up to the event. It's saying, 'No wonder I feel stressed or uneasy, it's the first day at my new job.' Normalising the situation removes uncertainty, substitutes it with clarity and puts you back in control. It's normal to feel a certain way at a certain time.

Using one or two words to describe an emotion can reduce its energy. This technique is called symbolic labelling. However, if you open up a full-blown conversation about an emotion, or stay with it, you will actually increase its power. If you hide it away, or try to suppress an emotion, it's always there, whereas giving it a name and moving on can remove its power. One of the most famous examples of this is Winston Churchill, who referred to his depressive episodes as his black dog. Giving them a name helped him come to terms with his disorders and the need for help with them.

It's all mindfulness related, being in tune with what's occurring. It's about being aware, paying attention with intention to the here and now with openness, acceptance and without judgement.

It's also about pressing pause. I now want to introduce you to a very special formula of life:

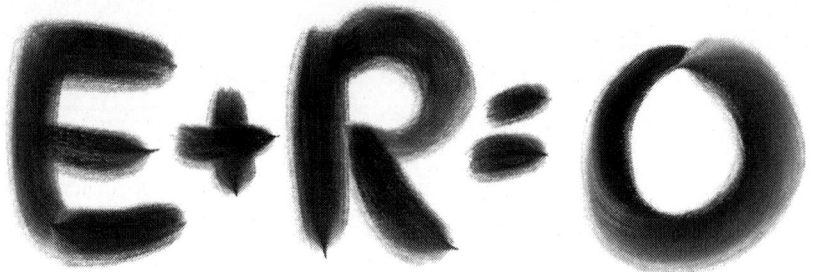

EVENT + RESPONSE = OUTCOME

I first discovered this formula in the book *Above the Line* by Urban Meyer, a hugely successful American football coach. The subtitle of his book is 'Lessons in leadership and life'. It's a brilliant book and one I regularly revisit, especially when coaching leaders and teams.

In the book he asks, 'How do you bring your best when it matters most?' That's a powerful question. He then references a simple but powerful equation that he says affects everything we do. The truth is that, since discovering this, I'm not sure I've gone many days without using it. His point is that we rarely control the events in our lives and don't directly control the outcomes – but we *can* choose and control how we respond.

So, the 'E' is any event, situation or circumstance that might occur in life. The 'R' is how we respond, and the 'O' is the outcome of that response. The theory being that if we are not entirely happy with the outcomes then we need to change the 'R', our response to such events. Once you get it, it becomes a magnificent tool with many benefits with the obvious being better outcomes.

An event could be anything from a sales call to your entire life. Basically, if you're not happy with the outcome then change your response. The responsive actions are our choice and what the formula does is push you to deciding what outcome you would like before you respond.

Furthermore, it helps you press pause and remove emotion keeping the 'R' to stand for response and not reaction! Urban says this is not easy and needs to be practised. He goes on to say that pressing pause gives you time to think, it gets you off autopilot and helps you gain clarity about the outcome you are pursuing. Isn't that just fantastic? Clarity is what we all seek and is the essential ingredient to making progress and achieving success.

Urban Meyer calls the response the 'R' factor and says this factor can determine the quality of your life. As I said, it's a magnificent tool if you incorporate it into your life. You can use it for almost anything. Try it as soon as possible. Just ask, 'What outcome do I want from this situation (the event)?' You have already pressed pause.

That's E+R=O.

When you become more expert at living in a mindful way, you will notice improvements in all your senses. Colours appear richer and brighter, food tastes better, your sense of smell is greater, and you pick up more surrounding sounds such as birds singing or the wind blowing.

You also develop into a brilliant listener, tuning in to various signals and emotions from the person you are in contact with. The conversation becomes more meaningful and of a higher quality and value. The other person will feed off and respond positively to intentional attention. It's a communication breakthrough when you become a great listener, I promise.

I persevered and practised and reached a point whereby I could spot a negative thought like a black cloud moving in from the distance. This enabled me to deploy my samurai to deal with these dark intruders well in advance. I began to live a more fulfilling life from then on, knowing I had that inside support and defence in place.

There is a superb poem by Robert Conklin called 'I am Your Master' that unpacks a thought, suggesting it can send you to the bright lights of success or the darkness of failure. It's from his book *Be Whole* and very cleverly written. The conclusion of the poem says that a thought can never be removed but it can be replaced. My interpretation is that we just need to understand and appreciate that it's just a thought but it has a spectrum of power. Our challenge is to control it and not let it control us.

Now think of this, we can deploy our samurai to fight of negativity, but now consider allowing our innate and mindful monk to help us find peace.

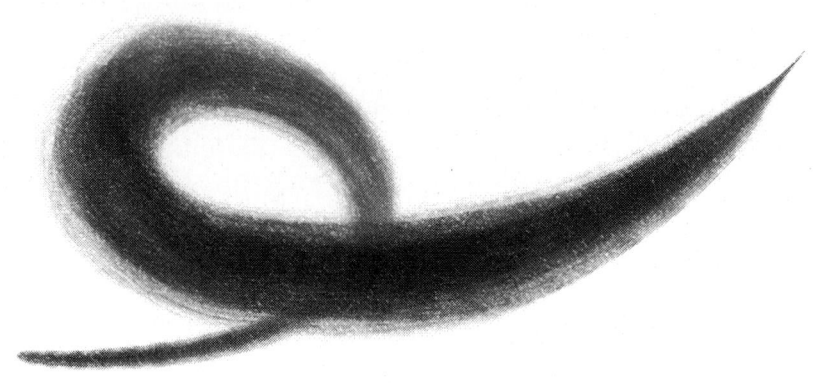

Mindfulness begins with breath. It's always there, it doesn't go away or have to be found. Breath is life and it's the anchor to mindful living. In truth, the breath is the most important lifeforce of all. We can go days without food and water but a few minutes without breathing. And, strangely, because we do it unconsciously, we take it for granted.

The main purpose of the breath is to supply the body and brain with enough oxygen to operate effectively. When we breathe quickly with shallow breaths the result is stress, tension and a muddled mind. Breath gives us an anchor for meditation because when we focus on it, it brings us back to the present moment.

Dr. Bhante Saranapala, lovingly known as The Urban Monk, talks about meditation being a healing technique. He says:

'Mindfulness meditation is an internal medicine for peace and well-being. When you are unwell and go to the doctor, the doctor gives you a prescription whereby you might take the medicine twice a day to recover. In the same way meditation must be taken.'

In martial arts and, in particular, the art I studied, Shotokan karate, the timing of breathing is similarly key. Every move made in martial arts has a well-timed inhalation and exhalation and this alone requires years of practice. In this case, timing of the breath is central to producing destructive power and is, therefore, fundamental in the relationship between the breath and an energy force referred to as *ki* or *chi*. On one side peace and serenity on the other devastating power. Breath is quite simply the anchor of life.

For your reference, *ki* is Japanese, and *qi* and *chi* are Chinese translations. *Ki* means many things such as air, mind, intention and will. It's said to be the unseen force, a universal energy that can be accessed. *Ki* is often translated as spirit or energy, and we will cover this in more detail in the purple belt syllabus.

The practice of mindfulness meditation revolves around the breath. It's the only certain way to anchor yourself in the present moment. When you focus on the breath there is nothing else but the here and now. By paying attention to each breath, you are released from your past and future. Introducing breathing meditations into your life alone will help reduce stress and anxiety, as well as providing many more benefits.

When we pay attention to our breath and breathing, we can achieve a state of calmness. It's our innate pause button too as deep focussed breathing activates our parasympathetic system, sometimes referred to as our 'rest and digest system' that I referenced in the yellow belt syllabus. When in play, the parasympathetic system's job is to calm the body down and lower the heart rate, allowing the body to increase digestion. In reality, it's opposing the sympathetic system which prepares our body to deal with stress and fear activating the fight or flight response we witnessed through the yellow belt grade.

I explained at the start of this syllabus that in martial arts we must be relaxed and calm but incredibly focussed. The state of peak performance and mindful breathing exercises, once developed into habits and meditations, form a regular, rich mental nourishment that really is one of the secret elixirs of life.

I need to reinforce how important it is to incorporate self-encouragement and self-compassion into our lives. Our samurai is there working closely with our monk providing calmness and moment-to-moment centred attention, while having the tools and weaponry to overthrow any attacks from our troublesome and, occasionally, punishing minds.

The last part of my learning, which again was significant in my own awakening, was the practice and understanding of reflection. Taking time to process situations, thoughts and feelings. Reflection is pressing pause with the aim of finding a clear and honest perspective but without making judgements. It's giving something careful consideration to obtain clarity. It's so helpful but does need a lot of work for it to become another layer of our personal protection system.

I end this syllabus with a quote. Good luck with your grading.

'You can search throughout the entire universe for someone who is more deserving of your love and affection than you are yourself, and that person is not to be found anywhere. You yourself, as much as anybody in the entire universe deserve your love and affection.' ~ BUDDHA

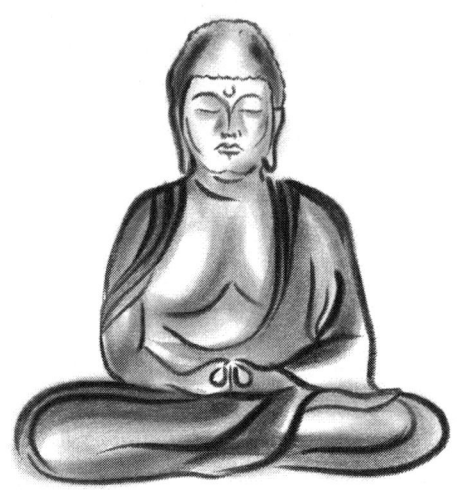

GREEN BELT GRADING WARM-UP:

This syllabus focussed on an ancient wisdom that emanated from Buddhism; mindfulness, something we all possess the ability to practise, and benefit from its life-changing components. Through the yellow belt grade, we unpacked the devastating results of the stealth-like killer, stress, and how mindfulness is the most wonderful intervention to combat suffering in both corrective and preventative courses of action. In a world of information overload mindfulness helps us to cut through it and centre ourselves.

We covered many elements of mindfulness and how it can translate into a way of living. It's about learning to spend less time in our past and future and more time in the present moment. It sounds simple but, like everything, if we want to get good at it, we need to practise.

Awareness is a skill that can be developed over time. The self-awareness part, the ability to focus on yourself is key. With practice, you can observe how your thoughts, emotions and reactions respond to certain situations. Becoming an observer to what's occurring is one thing but doing it without judgement is what delivers the best results. This is transformational learning, as once you begin to step out and tune in to what's happening in real time you can begin to make important adjustments to help control and regulate your thoughts and emotions. Another benefit is that being self-aware helps us recognise our strengths and weaknesses. Add to that the fact the awareness takes us outside of ourselves into a new world of appreciation of what surrounds us. Being acutely aware opens up to the outer world and brings with it advanced listening skills, empathy and the ability to observe nature in its true essence.

We looked at meditation, another ancient practice, and how breath is the anchor of life. When it becomes a routine or a ritual, meditation transitions into a mindful way of living. It's said that the most important moment of meditation is the moment you sit down to do it because you're saying, 'I care for myself.'

We tapped into the hardwired negative bias we possess to help us understand why our emotions are more powerful when we lose something versus gaining something and covered emotional tools such as normalising and labelling that help us deal with certain situations.

Apply yourself to this grading. Don't hold back, give it all you've got!

GREEN BELT GRADING

1. Read 'The Man in the Glass' again and note any further insights gained this time around.

2. Step outside of yourself and observe how you are feeling. Give yourself a check-over, your private and personal audit. Jot down your findings and, in particular, anything that stands out such as stress, tightness or how good you feel.

3. Your first official *Mokuso* meditation.

    - Find a place that you can relax in. It needs to be peaceful.

    - Take a seat that brings with it a sense of calmness or sit on the floor. You can kneel or sit cross-legged as long as you are comfortable.

    - Start at five minutes. Set your timer. Make sure your alarm sound is a soft reminder and not a police siren or the school bell.

    - Start to concentrate on your breath, breathing in and out.

    - To keep focussed and fixed in the moment start to count in for three seconds and out for four or even five. Please note a longer exhale than the inhale moves the nervous system away from stress activating the parasympathetic system.

    - Feel and observe the sensations of the breath in and out.

    - Gradually loose the conscious counting but keep focussed on the breath, keeping with that rhythm.

    - Notice when your mind has wandered and gently return your attention back to the breath bringing you back to the here and now.

    - Acknowledge any thoughts and don't judge yourself. Just ease the focus back to the breath.

    - To close your practice, convert your mindfulness to kindfulness and notice how you feel right now, your senses, your thoughts and emotions. And more than anything, please acknowledge that those five precious minutes were dedicated to you only. It was mindful me-time. Please note your experience in your book of life.

    - Aim to include this meditation as part of your daily routine just a few minutes to begin with. As time goes on, and you become more skilful and accustomed to your mindful meditation routine, increase your time to ten minutes. Try to complete at the start and at the end of every day. Remember your attention in this exercise has been anchored by your breath. In time, you can expand your practice with outside influences such as various sounds and sights, a candle, the sky, the trees and so on. Make this exercise into a habit; it's going to become a beautiful addition to your life.

4. Produce three key points that really grabbed your attention from this syllabus and remember to record everything in your journal.

Congratulations, my readers!
You are now a green belt.
Awesome work!

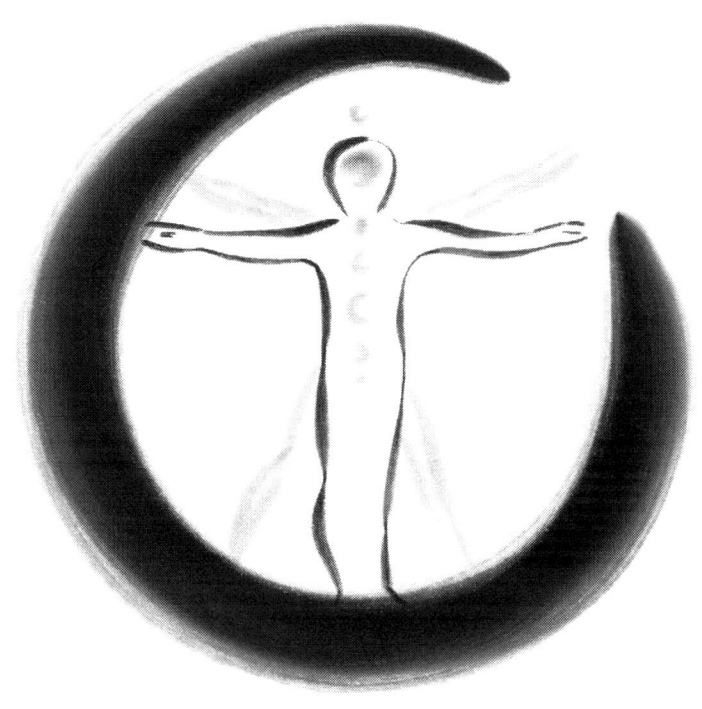

CHAPTER 6
PURPLE BELT
Mind and Body Mastery

'Mastering others is strength, mastering yourself is true power.'
~ LAO TZU

In ancient Chinese philosophy, yin and yang is about all things having two sides, two facets. They are neither good nor bad, or oppose or complement each other, but the two elements cannot exist without each other. In this syllabus I bring together the mind and body and the universal energy that connects the two to create a balanced, healthy, mindful and happy life. This is the way to a lifestyle of well-being; the secret to living a black belt life.

Your journey kitbag is now filling up with tools, weaponry and your inner compass to help navigate you along the way. As a green belt you discovered two spiritual inner masters in the form of the monk and the samurai. They defeat darkness and negativity and bring positivity, light, peace and calmness into your life. The monk and the samurai; our spiritual yin and yang.

This belt focuses on the body and management of your physical health and well-being. The purple belt syllabus will help you to understand and appreciate the physical aspects of life and ignite changes to your life journey. This is another crucial element to accelerate your progress through to black belt.

It's time to look, listen, respond.

We have worked hard on gaining an appreciation of the power of the mind and the spectrum of results it can produce. You have acquired life-enhancing psychological skills and can now fully appreciate the astonishing superpower of self-belief. You have gained vital techniques, tools and tactics to provide your brain with rich mental nourishment; brain food that fuels positivity! We have learned that inspiration leads to motivation which combats negative thinking and helps maintain mental control.

Now it's time to turn our attention back to the body and provide the balance needed to gain an appreciation of mind and body mastery. It's not what you think it is.

I named one of my public speaking events, 'The Gateway to Mind and Body Mastery'. I began by covering what mind and body mastery is not! I showed a slide containing photos of four different people; Albert Einstein, a Benedictine monk, an Olympic athlete and a world-famous footballer with his shirt off sporting a toned, defined and ripped physique.

My point was, you don't have to have the IQ of Einstein, the devout vows of the monk, or be an Olympic athlete or possess a body like a football god to achieve mind and body mastery. The gateway to mind and body mastery is the opening up and expanding of your awareness and attention towards it – your mind is the gateway. It's about mastering the skill of listening. You are learning to listen to your mind and to observe your thoughts. But it's equally important to pay close attention to what your body is telling you, then respond accordingly. We tend to violate the rules of the body, therefore, it's crucial we start to spend more quality time with it. It's not a consideration, it's a must-do.

Once they have unpacked their dreams and goals, I regularly say to my clients that to achieve them there is one crucial factor. It's you! Yes, you must get in shape, be in shape and stay in shape. You must look after yourself as without 'you' none of this works. Without you there can be no goals, no dreams and no success.

So, let's look at what getting in and staying in shape means!

WELLNESS

A wellness-focussed strategy is essential for any personal development journey as, without exception, every one of my clients discovers.

I want you to keep this in mind – your body is unique and needs a great deal of attention! Your body is not a car, you can't upgrade it as it gets old, if it keeps breaking down or if it starts to show a few dents and scratches. Your body is the only place you have to live! You might be able to move house if your home no longer serves your needs, but you can't move body. You have one body – therefore, it's important to show it respect.

Ask yourself: 'Do I want to feel better physically? Could I get fitter, walk further, cycle more, eat more healthily, hydrate more, be more interested in what I eat and when I eat it?' Surely the answer has to be YES! There is always something you can improve on.

In this syllabus we look at how to care for your body, maintain it and get the best out of it whatever its age, shape or condition right now. We will pay attention to the relationships between nutrition and fitness, a healthy diet and regular exercise, which all help towards living a long, healthy and happy life – a black belt life.

I'm not going to supply you with a black belt nutrition-focussed diet, or a black belt body-busting fitness and exercise regime that will transform your physique, size, strength and stamina in three months, three weeks or three days. No, this grading syllabus is designed to help you become more aware of your body, pay more attention to it and dial in to the energy it creates, maintaining the inside-out living philosophy. That continuous improvement ethos of personal growth helps you make smart decisions that will take you to another level of life. Some people joke about their body being a temple. Well, your body actually is your private, personal, unique shrine and it's time to start worshipping it.

I fully appreciate everyone is different and there are exceptions to the rule when it comes to what is the best way to look after yourself. Scientists often cite the previously referenced Winston Churchill as a good example of someone who effectively broke all the rules of maintaining a healthy lifestyle and made it to a good age. His cardiologist wrote, 'I'm amazed he made it to age ninety. He was fat, sedentary and stressed, he smoked cigars and drank alcohol to excess, and kept terribly irregular hours.' It is also said he suffered with dark moods, depression and despair, had little energy, spent a great deal of time in bed and, during his last ten years, suffered four strokes. Yes, he can be described as an exception to the rule in terms of his longevity but that's it. He most certainly did not live a black belt life. I wonder how much more he could have achieved or how much better he might have felt if he hadn't abused his body the way he did.

It's time to look at how we behave towards our bodies, how we fuel ourselves and keep our physical selves well-serviced.

I want to take you back to one of my earliest memories as a child. My mum is, at the time of writing this book, eighty-five years old. I can remember throughout my life, one of her favourite sayings to me and others was, 'everything in moderation'. This was her philosophy to well-being. So, I checked out the word 'moderation' and here are some of its synonyms: self-control, self-discipline, restraint and balance. These amazingly appropriate words partly sum up not only this chapter, but the entire journey of the way. For this belt they must all be directed at how you manage your body. They all appear in the 'One Word' survey at the start of this book.

In a nutshell, my mum's personal philosophy is supported by the ancient Greek physician Hippocrates, referred to as the 'Father of Medicine'. He said, *'If we could give every individual the right amount of nourishment and exercise, not too little and not too much, we would have found the safest way to health.'*

Mum, your theory is also backed by today's science, particularly when focussing on the enhancement and maintenance of a healthy lifestyle. Brilliant, Mum! Just brilliant!

We discovered in the orange belt that we can develop amazing mental muscle by building a strong and powerful belief structure. This becomes our core mindset, a solid centre of mental strength oozing self-confidence and self-worth with a clear goal-setting capacity. Our physical core is equally meaningful. Technically, it comprises the abdominal muscles, pelvis and lower back. People with a weak core generally suffer with lower back pain, poor posture and sometimes shortness of breath. Our core is also positioned where our vital organs do a great deal of work and where some of our largest and most important veins and arteries are based. Therefore, strong core muscles help support this part of our operating system, too.

Many of us find ourselves sitting for long periods with an arched back and tilted pelvis. We get stiff and lethargic and get used to an aching back and shoulders and headaches. This pain becomes normal to us, an everyday occurrence; we accept it as part of our life.

In karate training we focus fundamentally on the technical side, building and honing a specific and special set of skills. However, to be in a condition to execute those skills, the exercise and training, fitness planning, stretching drills and so on must take place outside the dojo in your own time. In martial arts it's the training and practice you do outside the dojo that takes you to black belt, so the third and fourth pillars of the way are paramount – 'commitment and discipline'.

In the beginning of the way I challenged and opened up your thinking, your awareness and redirected your focus. Now I'm going to stretch you further, but in the physical sense. I could not believe how from a stiff and broken cricketer I transformed into someone who could comfortably deliver a devastating kick to a person's head, even if they were over 6 feet tall. With control of course! Yes, I had to master the technique through perseverance and repetition, but it was the continuous flexing and stretching of my body that eventually allowed me to execute those moves.

A few minutes stretching each day, every day, can become life-changing for anyone and everyone. Firstly, it is about identifying the target areas, finding out what works and building new habits into your lifestyle, even just for a few minutes a day. You can combine habits too, for example when you stretch you can meditate, and clear your head at the same time. It's a win-win.

If you're concerned about your health and/or fitness, then a sensible starting point would be checking-in with your GP to arrange a professional health check and then build from there. Always seek advice from your GP or qualified personal trainer before you start any form of physical exercise. Once you've sought expert guidance, take time out to research a stretching plan that works with your body.

Remember though, you need to *stay* in shape to make this all happen. I make no apologies in repeating that without you there is no achievement. It doesn't matter how old you are, what shape you're currently in, if you are a member of a gym or not, if you have a high-performing wellness/fitness-based lifestyle or not, don't worry, this syllabus will help you improve from this point on. Your starting point is now.

So, what's the first thing we are going to do?

As always, we're going to begin with awareness; with becoming more mindful of what you consume, how you exercise, rest, relax and recharge.

Let's work on feeling physically healthier by improving your fitness levels and introducing small changes to your wellness habits that will produce dramatically impactful results. Inactivity itself has been described by the UK Department of Health as 'the silent killer'. Stress has also been described using the same words. In short you must keep moving.

I don't really need to drive home the countless benefits of physical exercise, such as reducing the risk of major illness including cancer, heart disease, type 2 diabetes and lowering the risk of depression and early death.

Top athletes speak about their physical fitness fuelling their mental capacity to keep driving forward. This outlines the incredible interlinked relationship between mind, body and soul, and how when all of them are aligned in harmony, there is an opportunity to achieve exponential growth and to experience greater fulfilment. It's all to do with how they work together.

It's the same as the relationship between self-esteem and self-efficacy. If you do something well, it makes you feel good and raises your self-esteem. When your self-esteem is high you tend to do things well, which improves your self-efficacy and so on.

When exercising, your body sets off a series of chemical reactions. You already know what happens in the fight or flight response from your progress though the yellow belt syllabus. While regular exercise won't produce the same reaction, some interesting neurochemistry will occur making the experience an enjoyable and rewarding one.

I now know why I always felt so magnificent when leaving the dojo and why I was totally pumped and buzzing during the journey home in the car. When my daughter started training with me, even at a young age, you could tell she was also on a high when we got into the car together. Feeling such a rush, drowning in a sea of adrenaline, we used to crank the music up playing 'The Chain' by Fleetwood Mac and 'You & Me' by The Wannadies, time and time again. The 'You and Me' song, by the way, is still 'our song' to this day. Marvellous, heart-warming memories and I'm so pleased I can share them with you.

We were experiencing another 'D.O.S.E.' of the same neurotransmitters referenced in the orange belt syllabus. A cocktail of dopamine and serotonin that led to a feeling of pulsating excitement. And this is just the start of the extensive list of benefits from a physical workout.

When I revisit the story of 'The Amazing Fred' in the green belt chapter, I realise that the gym was my go-to when I felt low, stressed, sad or worse during that difficult time. It was like a magnet to me. I was drawn to it and, in truth, I used to smash myself on the bike and cross trainer. It reached the point where I could have gone on forever on the cross trainer. I think, sadly, it was because I didn't want those negative emotions to return and I was feeding off the endorphins. I didn't want the happy cocktail to wear off.

With your belief structure in place and some amazing tools in your life kitbag, it's very important to start to visualise how your life will be transformed with a new focus on feeling fitter, sharper, stronger, more energetic and generally much healthier. This is the continuation of the self-discovery experience of the way.

I have one of my own quotes on my coaching website:

'Self-discovery is when untapped potential is unearthed then unleashed and is one of the most motivational things a human being can experience.' ~ PHIL TOOGOOD

I'm living proof of this, as are my clients and millions of other people. When you discover something new about yourself or when you develop something you already have and take it to greater levels, it's an unbelievable feeling.

Many years ago, I had to stop running as a pastime due to Achilles' injuries. So, I turned to cycling. Being a sportsman over so many years and someone who relentlessly gave 100% I spent a great deal of my time injured. I learnt quickly that if one part of my body was out of action then there would be many other areas I could work on.

Strangely, I worked with a client using that exact same philosophy. While his injury was healing through rest and physiotherapy, he developed other areas of his body and mind, utilising his time wisely and effectively. By the time his injury had healed, he was stronger, fitter and sharper.

We can apply this example of creative thinking to many aspects of our life. Instead of dwelling on a problem and sinking into a sea of negativity, we can design new ways and thinking styles to create a different outlook. This is a powerful message I want you to take away from this syllabus. Never give up, use the fifth pillar of the way – perseverance. There will always be something you can do.

Marcus Aurelius said, *'Reject your sense of injury and the injury itself disappears.'*

When I took up cycling, to reduce the impact to both of my Achilles, I bought bikes that were conducive to summer and winter cycling. I discovered a whole new world, a new experience. Not only did cycling improve and maintain my fitness levels, I reached a point whereby my greatest insights and creativity arrived when I was cycling in the countryside. It was, and still is, one of the most wonderful and rewarding things I do, and again I discovered this late on in my life.

I realise how fortunate I am to live in rural England. I am blessed on my journeys to often feel at one with nature, experiencing the different seasons and the changes they bring with them; the landscape, colours, smells, wildlife and birds singing. I often stop to watch deer in the field or crossing the roads. On numerous occasions I have tried to capture an amazing landscape or the sun setting by taking a photo using my phone, because sometimes, when you are in the moment, it's quite emotional and you get the urge to share the experience. I am, at these times, experiencing mindfulness in its purest form, it's a feeling of enlightenment on the inside, while looking at something wonderful on the outside. No camera in the world can capture that, only your memory.

At times the experience is quite overwhelming and, although difficult to describe, the best explanation would be to say I feel completely dialled into life. It's a beautiful feeling. Why I share this with you is to help you appreciate that there are many untapped hidden wonders you can benefit from by making just one change to your life. I decided to ride a bike for fitness reasons and my life changed for many other reasons, not just my fitness. I found a perfect space in which to centre myself, discover nature and, at times, I have been awash with spontaneous insights, ideas and creativity.

So, let's look at your physical well-being. Ask yourself some further questions.

Am I getting out of puff climbing the stairs or walking the dog? What and where are my aches and pains? Am I going to put up with them or attempt to do something positive about them? Do I want to push myself a little further? And, ultimately, what am I prepared to do to live a black belt life?

Once again, it's time to deploy the monk and the samurai.

Many people find conversations relating to personal habits such as eating fast or processed food, smoking, drinking alcohol and so on, immensely challenging. This is because they have become so habitual. No one likes to admit they have bad habits, so when spoken about, it usually takes them immediately into threat and self-justification mode. They withdraw and/or get defensive, making excuses for their actions. I have seen it so many times, especially when it comes to smoking, body weight and general fitness.

Most smokers you meet will openly admit that smoking is bad for them. The majority clearly state they should give up, and they want to give up. They have made many attempts to quit and, usually, state categorically that they will give up in the future. You can sense an awkwardness, a sort of anxiety from the person as they continue to justify their reasons for not quitting.

Many people treat body weight in the same way. You tend to hear the same narrative – 'I know I'm overweight and could do with losing a few pounds. I know I would benefit in so many ways, I must start walking more, running, cycling, going to the gym, changing my diet, cutting down on alcohol, drinking more water.' But they do nothing about these concerns because they are the result of deeply embedded habits.

I had a client who refused to get on the scales as he didn't want to see his weight. This mindset stemmed from one occasion, when on a fitness improvement programme, he put on a pound in weight after hours of training and changes to his diet, nutrition and hydration. We know this sometimes happens with health programmes, with the loss of fat and gain in muscle, but it destroyed him and, subsequently, he was against using scales as a measurement of progress. He would rather use his belt buckle as the indicator.

By working on his mindset, he flipped the negativity into a positive outlook and embraced what the figures showed. Remember they are just numbers, and we addressed the fact that it's how you choose to process them, either as a negative and demotivational driver or as a positive influence and motivational opportunity. Our response is a choice, our choice and this mindset when understood becomes a breakthrough moment for people. Thinking is a choice, and can become a pattern, a habit. Remember, we can start new thinking habits which drive new actions.

Do you gain a pound and quit? Or do you gain a pound and grow more determined? You're the only one who can choose which path you take, and you can use your experience and knowledge of goal setting that you acquired as a red belt. If you apply this process, then you are guaranteed success. If you want me to tell you it's easy, well, I'm not going to. Change is tough, whether it's mind or body. But it's our attitude that makes the difference between success and failure.

The truth is, when I write this, I'm thinking to myself how absurd this is because essentially this should be the easy part of the journey as, in most societies, we are educated to a relatively high standard as to what is good for us and what is not. We know the answers and clearly understand the way to healthier living. Again, it's translating the words, the thinking, into 'doing'.

Eleanor Roosevelt said, *'No one can make you feel inferior without your consent.'* It's the same philosophy you should approach these situations with. Embrace them, set a mental filter or deploy the samurai to defeat any negative thought responses. Remember it's about mindset.

I'm now going to make it even easier for you.

As I've said, martial arts is a continual learning experience from white to black, with a never-ending culture of learning and development. You learn a move in weeks then spend years or, potentially, the rest of your life refining it. In order to do this, we keep reverting to the fundamentals. In karate we take it right back to the basics; how we breathe, our stance and posture, move and focus. The same philosophy can be applied to the way we live our life.

For body mastery we do not need to invest in state-of-the-art equipment, revolutionary new technologies for fitness and well-being, nor the millions of diet or exercise programmes that promise to deliver fast results and energy levels along with the body of an athlete with an abdominal six pack. This grade is about assessing what you are currently doing and cultivating a new and mindful way of improving your current personal health and well-being. They key word is 'current'.

To strengthen my point, may I introduce you to Charles Atlas, born in 1892, an Italian-born, American bodybuilder. He won titles such as the 'World's Most Perfectly Developed Man'. It is said he was a skinny and weak boy and took beatings from neighbourhood bullies and his uncle. Growing up he became inspired by the statue of Hercules and a lion and tiger he saw in the Bronx Zoo. He thought about how these animals remain in perfect condition. He watched them flex and stretch and saw their huge, shapely muscles standing out from their lean bodies.

Determined to get fit and change his physique, but too poor to purchase a set of barbells, Charles went on to invent a system called 'dynamic tension' based on isometric exercises, using zero equipment. Pushing one arm against another in different ways, squats, sit-ups and leg lifts – with the help of fitness writer, Dr Frederick Tilney, he went on to patent The Dynamic Tension Program, which quickly went on to become hugely popular. Some of the most famous names in sporting history took on the program, such as heavyweight boxing champion Rocky Marciano, Joe Lewis and Allan Wells who won the 1980 Moscow Olympic Games 100-metre gold medal.

Now I have made you aware of Charles's incredible story, I hope he has inspired you, because he is evidence that there is always a way. No excuses!

There is a saying, 'Keep doing what works, stop doing what doesn't and try something new'. You might have shaped the way you are over time, but the most astonishing thing is that you can reshape and recondition yourself using the power of the mind first. We humans have this astonishing capability to create change to our mental health, mindset, mental capacity, physical fitness and overall well-being and outlook. You have the power; you have the tools. It's within your control, start now, you only have one body.

Regularly remind yourself of the underpinning philosophy of this book, and that is living life from the inside out. Focussed self-awareness is required throughout your journey. Therefore, it is critical that you take time to listen to your body as well as your mind, they will tell you everything so pay attention to them. Your body will tell you exactly how you are and thus guide you to invest time and resources into fixing or improving it.

So, are you feeling tired – do you need more rest? Is your sleep pattern poor – do you need to learn how to relax and wind down? Are you feeling lethargic – should you be exercising more to boost your energy levels? If your shoes were pinching your feet, you'd pay attention to the pain and change your shoes. Think about that for a moment.

With my coaching clients, early on in the process, I reference the first pillar – honesty. Honesty from the get-go is the starting point that allows us to be able to measure progress as we move forward. Being honest creates the benchmark. I ask all my clients to read the poem 'The Man in the Glass' just as you have done throughout your gradings.

To move forward, set new goals, change your lifestyle and put a greater onus on wellness within your day-to-day life structure you need to start with honesty. The question is, where am I now and where would I like to be?

A LIFE IN BALANCE

Just for a short while I'd like to focus on one word that means moderation – 'balance'. In martial arts training balance is critical. Why? To be able to produce immense power with a kick or a punch or to avoid attack with split second response times. Our core is where our physical power is stored, and balance helps your stability and, therefore, your control. For this reason, great gymnasts have amazing core strength. Developing our physical core is the most important element of achieving good balance.

I had to work very hard on my balance for karate. My determination to improve it became an obsession to a point I used to brush my teeth in the morning and at night standing on one leg. I often found myself standing on one leg while waiting for someone, or talking on the phone. I tried to do it covertly, lifting my leg a few inches off the ground so it wasn't noticeable to people walking past me. I eventually mastered it. How? It goes right back to the title of the white belt chapter – 'attitude is everything'. It's attitude that gets you where you want to go or how high you want to travel. In the words of Zig Ziglar, *'Your attitude determines your altitude.'* To what

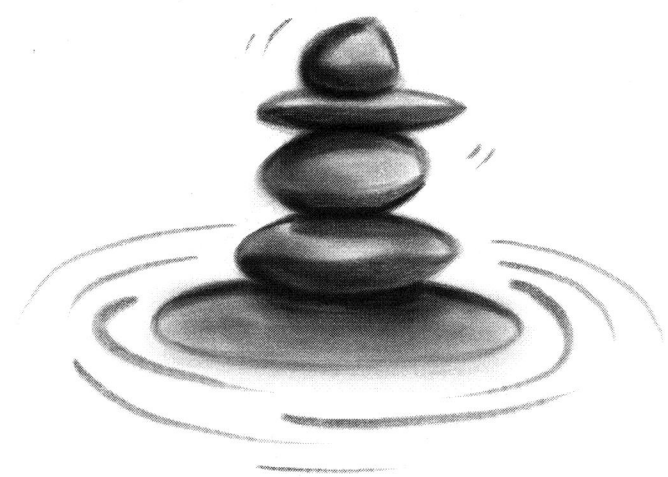

new heights will your new black belt attitude take you?

A commonly used phrase these days is work-life balance. It's something we cannot ignore as, essentially, it's about balancing our lives. From the outside in – our work, our social life and being active. From the inside out, it is finding some peace and quietness, checking-in with ourselves. Strangely with most of us what's needed is more time spent on looking inwards, more me-time to identify and initiate that critical balance. When our lives are out of balance, as many are, everything gets out of kilter. One of the areas that tends to suffer most is diet and exercise.

A report published by the UK National Health Service (NHS) in May 2020, evaluating 2018-19 data, stated that during that twelve-month period 876,000 hospital admissions reported obesity as a factor. An increase of 23% from the previous year. It also concluded that 20% of Year 6 children were categorised as obese – that's one in five! But also, the majority of adults were overweight or obese. That's 67% men and 60% of women. Now, I appreciate there can be many factors that lead to becoming overweight such as genetics, medication and brainwashing by the media and marketeers, however, these mind-blowing statistics are largely down to bad eating habits and a lack of exercise.

The diet and weight-loss industry has grown globally into a multi-billion-dollar market. There are thousands of books and programmes that claim to be the best, the most impactful and the most beneficial for us as humans. The truth is, the reason why libraries are full of books on this topic, is because there is not one universal magical system out there that guarantees success for everyone. If it did exist, we would all be using it and the others would be in the recycling bin.

Whichever 'system' works for you – it all comes down to balance. To maintain a healthy weight, we must balance the calories (energy) in against the calories (energy) out. It honestly is that simple. Doing this by fuelling your body with a well-balanced, nutritious diet is, of course, more beneficial, but everyone's requirements are unique and driven by their lifestyle. Elite athletes require additional energy to fuel their performance. Bodybuilders require protein rich diets to build their muscles. Endurance athletes require slow-release energy to provide continued fuel.

With so many 'diets' sold to us through so many mediums it can be confusing. But what if you forget the word 'diet' and replace it with 'lifestyle'? A diet gives the impression of something that starts and stops when you have achieved your goal. But if you stop – what will happen? If you revert to bad habits, you will begin to gain weight again. Whereas, if you approach what you eat as how you choose to power your body and your well-being, it should become a continuous process of healthy living. An essential ingredient to a black belt life!

To be in balance, we also need to view treats that way too – a treat isn't a treat if it's something you have all the time. Find a healthy balance that allows you to enjoy your food and indulge occasionally. As my mum said, 'Everything in moderation.'

One other thing I feel I need to mention is hydration; we must watch our hydration habits as it's more than likely you need to hydrate more than you currently do. Water makes up two-thirds of our body and is, therefore, an essential vehicle that carries and directs nutrients, oxygen and glucose to various areas of the body. It helps with our natural waste system and lubricates our eyes and joints, and keeps our skin looking good. Do you know that if you feel thirsty and fancy a drink you are actually experiencing dehydration?

Headaches, lethargy, lack of concentration, mood changes and dizziness can be the consequences of low hydration levels. Also, weight gain and muscle cramps. The safest and most effective way to hydrate is with water as many fizzy drinks, squashes and juices contain added sugar.

In an article published by *Medical News Today* it says that the amount of water we drink depends on age and activity levels. That makes a lot of sense. Be mindful of your water intake. Review it, research it and I'm guessing you'll be upping your intake levels.

Once you have all this in place it's about building from that platform to suit your life requirements. If you exercise more then you will need more of the right fuel for your engine. Basically, you will need to tailor your programme to suit your lifestyle. I know it sounds easier than it is, but the skills you have learnt so far will help you map out your goals and go on to achieve them.

THE POWER OF HABIT

Our lives are made up of habits, some experts say that 95% of what we do is habitual! Good and bad. The secret to transcendence is not focussing on stopping old habits but creating new ones. It's amazing how this works when you understand the neuroscience behind it.

A habit is a particular set of neural connections and circuitry that has developed over time. The longer the habit, the more entrenched it becomes. It's an action or behaviour that we do automatically or subconsciously such as riding a bike, driving a car and brushing our teeth. Once we understand the task, do it correctly and then repeat it time and time again, it transitions to being automatic, and the mental energy needed to perform it reduces dramatically as the actions are moved to a different part of the brain.

The PFC in the brain is engaged first. As referenced in the yellow belt syllabus the neural part of the way, the PFC, is responsible for thinking and conscious decision-making. Scientists have discovered that any new task or activity triggers neurons, the brain's nerve cells, to fire up which start to create patterns or maps over time. The more the task is repeated the more embedded the pattern becomes both in the brain and in our behaviour. In 1949, Donald Hebb, a neuropsychologist, used the phrase 'neurons that fire together, wire together'.

What this means is that you have the unique ability to change your own brain and keep developing it, year in year out! It's called 'neuroplasticity'. In fact, it's called 'self-directed neuroplasticity'. The brain has the astonishing ability to adapt and change in response to new interactions within an environment. When we learn something new, we create new neural connections. When we learn something, new physical changes occur in our neural circuitry. Norman Doidge, psychiatrist and author says:

'Neuroplasticity is like snow. The first time you ski in fresh snow you can take any path you want as long as nothing is in the way. If it's a good run, you keep to the tracks for the next run and the next deepening the tracks, which become more difficult to get out of.'

This is exactly how the brain works in creating new habits through repetition that deepen and become more embedded neural pathways. So why not start something new and grow and strengthen some new neural circuitry. A word of warning though, the same thing applies to new 'bad' habits too, so choose wisely!

There are so many amazing examples of the miracle of neuroplasticity, such as stroke recovery and recovery from brain injuries. When a function is lost or damaged in one area of the brain, another area picks it up and starts to develop it. Isn't that incredible?

This should give you even more confidence and inner belief that anything is possible. Change is truly possible for all of us, whatever our age. We can learn new skills and grow as people, it's a divine gift that many of us are unaware of. Therefore, creating a new lifestyle is possible, and so is living a black belt life.

Remember, always approach change as something from which you will gain. This is a key learning point for this entire journey. Designing new routines and habits to bring about change must be viewed in terms of the benefits, as opposed to what you are losing or sacrificing. This psychology was behind the incredible success of the book *The Easy Way to Stop Smoking* by Allen Carr, who helped millions of people from all over the world give up smoking without the aid of drugs or other interventions.

At this stage, it is necessary to reinforce that living a black belt life is not about helping you to redesign your body, mind and spirit to superhuman levels. Yes, with parts of the journey's elements you will feel like you have acquired a few superpowers for sure, but it's about helping you find your hidden secret codes and inner guidance to transition to a healthier, happier and more fulfilling life. The black belt way is about discovering a new way to experience life. You can live life by design, you can make subtle but impactful changes, and, above all, you can learn and develop no matter who you are, where you are or how old you are.

YOGA

Other than martial arts, for me, the best way to achieve core strength, improve physical balance and posture, and make a transformational change to your overall wellness, is through yoga. Yoga focuses on various exercise poses and stretches, flexibility and breathing to boost core, physical and mental strength. Practising yoga has extraordinary benefits.

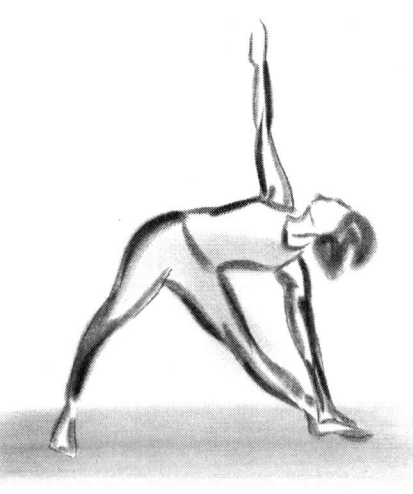

After bowing for the first time and entering the dojo, one of the most significant improvements I made to my life over time was my flexibility. Through twenty-five years of cricket, I was jammed up in my lower back, hips and hamstrings. I was determined to be able to perform some of the amazing kicks and move combinations that you learn to execute in karate. I applied the same principle to stretching as I did to developing my balance. Whereas, for a while, I spent a lot of my time on one leg to improve my balance, I selected a few key stretches, one in particular, and I would do them any chance I got – at work, an airport, the cinema – anywhere I could sit down. I found that I could convert the stretch slightly, so no one really knew what I was doing. Basically, it's about getting into a position that stretches out your hip flexors (at the top of your thighs) and your gluteus maximus (the muscles in your bum). These make up the largest muscle group in your body and are attached to your hips, pelvis, lower back and legs. When these are tight, they pull on both your lower back, like a sciatic type of pain, upper legs causing tight hamstrings, pelvic pain and even affect the knees. This exercise changed everything for me.

At the time I discovered the stretch, I had no idea it's referred to as the 'seated pigeon pose' in yoga. You can do it with or without a chair. It was so good I introduced this into the pre-match stretching for the cricket team I was coaching at the time, too. I never realised how stiff these young guys were around the lower back and hamstring area. Thinking about it, my brother-in-law, who graced some of the world's most famous football grounds with his speed and skills couldn't touch his toes as he was constantly stiff around his lower back and hamstrings. He often mentions that he wished he'd discovered yoga in those days as it might have extended his playing career or even improved his speed, capabilities and recovery while playing at an elite level.

When I reflect on the way to living a black belt life, most of the journey's hypothesis dates back thousands of years. Think about it; martial arts, mindfulness and philosophy, but all strongly supported by modern science. Now I add yoga, a practice that can be traced back a long way. Some researchers believe that it might be up to 10,000 years old, but it can certainly be traced to northern India 5,000 years ago. Incredible!

This ancient practice focuses on breathing and flexibility, which results in a plethora of mental and physical benefits. It's incredible how many ways yoga can improve your life. In martial arts we stretch and meditate, only for a few minutes at a time, but the combination of the two produce extraordinary outcomes.

It's said that there are nineteen different types of yoga and sixty-six basic yoga postures. Yoga has now been adapted for people of all ages and physical abilities and has become part of everyday life for many people.

I was lucky to experience the benefits of yoga taught by my local yoga teacher. The sessions lasted for about one hour and always ended in a lying position with candles burning and soft music playing in the background. She then went round to each person and covered them in a fleece blanket.

It was an amazing end to the session, and I used to drift off into another world. I do remember waking up on more than one occasion and for a split second, not having a clue where I was. When I left the session, I again experienced the feeling of being alive – a sensation of wellness that is difficult to describe.

Connecting slow, physical movement with our breath is another example of mindfulness in its purest form. It frees the mind and body, which is exactly why you feel so good, so refreshed and cleansed afterwards. It's mind and body utopia.

Early in the journey we focussed on stretching the mind, taking ourselves outside of our place of comfort into the field of learning. A fantastic quote depicts this perfectly:

'The comfort zone is a beautiful place, but nothing grows there.'
~ UNKNOWN

We must cultivate the same attitude towards our bodies too, as both need to be exercised regularly and cared for to maintain health and well-being.

SLEEP, REST AND REFRESH

As part of your life management there is a need to regularly check in and risk assess yourself, as referred to in the green belt syllabus, to identify if there are any challenging areas that need attention. A good way to describe this 'must-do' is as a kind of personal audit. Top of the list to evaluate is the cornerstone of life and performance. Sleep! So much research has been dedicated to sleep and why we need it. Scientific research has produced a great deal of evidence, particularly in recent times, to prove that it's impossible to consistently perform at our best without enough quality sleep. Books have been written on this subject so I will not go into too much detail here. But yes, it's clear, sleep is critical to performance. It's a process that is essential for optimum health.

Many people eat into their sleep as a part of their personal time management structure. The sleep window is often sacrificed for work-related duties. So many people are pushing to get more done and use what should be their sleep time to find extra hours. The consequences are brutal. Time management has become the devil in many people's lives. I have helped several clients with their time management, while continuously working to improve my own.

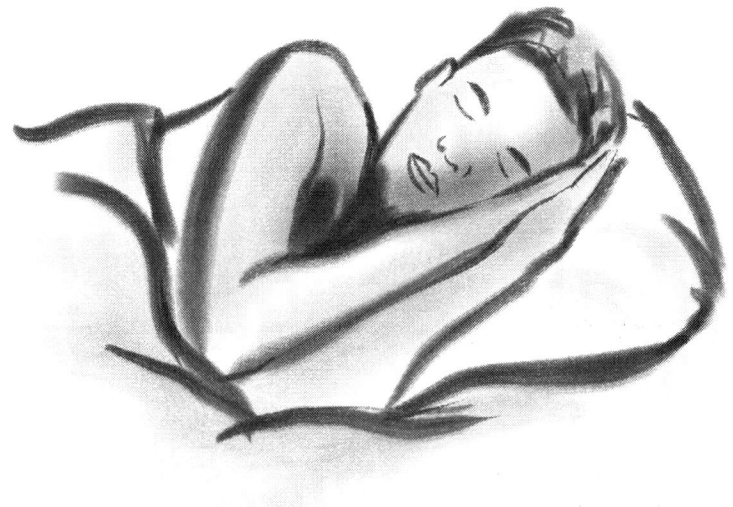

I have developed a theory that time is like an amazing, precious and magical pie. And because of its value, there needs to be a profitable return for each slice you give of it. The pie of time should be treated as a priceless asset and giving it away or investing it into something needs to generate a positive outcome. With this mindset you will be less flighty and wasteful of it. This creates the attitude that your investment of time at work or playing with your children returns equal measures of profit. Risk assess your pie of time. Spending time helping others should bring wonderful rewards as would going to the gym, meditating or reading a book in peace and quiet. Look at your time as a resource. We all have the same amount so just calculate how you can get the best from it.

The brain needs you to sleep. It doesn't stop, though, as it continues working hard to maintain its ultimate function in keeping you alive. It also prepares for your next day. It continues to work tirelessly filing information which, in turn, helps learning and memory banking.

The list of benefits and effects of having a good sleeping pattern is immense. It gives you a greater level of attention, you make less errors and mistakes, you're sharper, you learn more, become more creative and can make clearer decisions.

Studies have shown that the opposite occurs with a lack of sleep as it affects some areas of the brain. Sleep deficiency, along with poor problem-solving, bad decision-making and a lack of creativity, also affects emotional control and behaviour and has been linked to depression.

Sleep plays a vital role in the brain's ability to function and it needs between seven to nine hours a night for you to be at your best. Look at it this way, it's not 'you' that needs it, it's your brain. Looking after your brain will help you raise your game to perform at your best.

Think about it, throughout history sleep deprivation has been used as torture. Now analyse how you have felt and performed on your sleep quota. I'm yet to meet anyone who said they feel worse with more sleep.

I have worked with clients who really struggled with their sleep. Finding small or dramatic improvements to their sleep brought with it the confidence to achieve anything. Some had felt it was years since they had a good night's sleep.

Me, well, to be honest, I worked hard on myself to find the right balance that suited me. But, like most people, I have suffered a tremendous amount of lost sleep due to my thinking. No banging doors or loud music…just the noise and chatter in my head. I once went two days without sleep and that was a shocker, and this was on holiday! After that experience I suffered a mini phobia of going to bed and lying awake.

I have subsequently designed a sleep system that works for me. One of the main contributors to my success is that I always look for a positive and a gratitude that's occurred during my day. This helps me hit the pillow with a smile, and a smile is, for me, is the most important factor of all.

There are many sleeping tips and techniques out there; a good mattress and pillow, a blacked-out room and at least a thirty minutes' downtime from TV, smartphones, tablets and computers before you go to bed.

Meditation, using our method of *Mokuso* will help enormously and, again, there is science to support how meditation helps sleep. The reduction of stress and anxiety, calming the mind and connecting the mind and body together.

That's sleep covered but please be mindful of including rest in your life paradigm.

My meaning of rest is totally different to that of sleep. It's vital that rest is incorporated into your way of living. One definition of rest is 'the allowance to be inactive in order to regain strength or health'. Another says 'freedom from activity or labour'. Do you truly and deliberately make time to rest?

We might well notice our mind and body telling us we are tired and could do with a rest, but we tend to override our innate alarm bells and tap into any potential rest time to find more work and living space. However, ignore rest at your peril! Sometimes, we are just not aware that we need to rest until our mind and body demands it by shutting us down. Remember, this is what happened to 'The Amazing Fred' in the green belt syllabus. So, what does rest really look like?

My interpretation of rest is downtime, quite literally 'time down'. Yoga, meditation, mindful walking, hiking, cycling, exercise or gym work. It's all of the above or none of the above, it's about taking a break from your life agenda. It's *not doing* something as opposed to *doing* something. It's resting.

Rest could include reading a book or, perhaps, simply daydreaming, which used to be frowned upon by schoolteachers being judged as showing a lack of concentration and having a wandering mind. I can clearly remember being caught looking out of the window in a maths class. Yes, the truth is I was daydreaming. The teacher spotted me and the consequences were not good to say the least. And that's why I still, to this day, remember that event so clearly.

However, in today's busy world there is a place for daydreaming. Drifting off into another world far away from our inner and outer worlds, stretching into a new galaxy or frequency of existence can actually return positive results. It opens up a gateway to insights and invites creativity while switching off the cacophony of life's orchestra. According to Harvard University's health blog the wandering mind can help manage anxiety. Like meditation, daydreaming acts as a natural remedy to counter stress and can revitalise you.

An article published on the Verywell Mind (an information resource on mental health) website, says, *'Daydreaming has gotten a bad rap for too long! If you're stuck or frustrated or in need of some imagination and creativity give daydreaming a try and see what mental pathways might open up for you.'*

We now know that to lead a black belt life we have ancient practices available that will revitalise us, empty our cups and allow us to find that freshness, zest and vitality in the form of mindfulness, *Mokuso* meditation, yoga and more. These are all beautiful methods to enhance your health and well-being. But please find time to zone out and take a break.

One of the greatest stories relating to taking a break concerns one of the most famous breakthroughs and accomplishments in history. It occurred on 6th May, 1954, Roger Bannister breaking the four-minute mile.

Bannister was from a working-class family. Realising his talent for running, growing up, he won a track scholarship with Oxford University.

He competed in the 1500 metres in the 1952 Olympics, coming fourth. Disappointed with this result, he considered quitting running. Interestingly, his mental processing of this race flipped the potential negative outcome to a positive one and he used this disappointment as an incentive to drive him to his limits.

Breaking the holy grail of athletics, the four-minute mile was a historic and global quest for the world's best runners dating back to the ancient Greek Olympics as far as the eighth century BC. Greek folklore recounts some surprising methods to motivate runners to improve speed, such as lions being unleashed to chase the runners.

Moving forward into the twentieth century, the race attracted huge crowds but they never witnessed the four-minute mile being broken. A record time of four minutes and one second existed for close to a decade, through the 1940s into the 1950s.

It's believed that some expects felt that a sub four-minute mile was literally outside human capabilities. They felt that the body, especially the lungs and heart, would not withstand the punishment and impact in being pushed to that extent. Even death was a discussed as a consideration.

Roger chose an official race event at the Oxford University cinder track to attempt the record and try to break the unbreakable barrier. He got into perfect physical shape and condition using, at the time, new scientific methods studying the mechanics of running.

Then he did something that astonished many. He stopped training two weeks before the event! He decided to take a rest and went hiking and climbing in Scotland with friends. He said he felt stale but later admitted his decision was 'bordering on lunatic'. When he returned he continued to rest for another three days and, leading up to the event, just did some basic training.

So, before attempting to conquer what was described as 'humanly impossible' Roger decided to take a break for rest and recuperation. Absolutely incredible!

It was said that to run the perfect race the conditions needed also to be perfect. No wind and no rain. On the 6th May, they were the opposite with rain and a 25-mph crosswind blowing across the track. Bannister considered pulling out of the event but the wind dropped before the race was scheduled to begin. It had been carefully planned by Bannister and his coach that he would be aided by two pacemakers.

With 3,000 nervous spectators packed into the arena it was 6.00 pm when the starting gun was fired and the field of six went with Bannister tucked into second place. With three laps completed Bannister knew he was outside the sub four-minute time. The bell rang for the final lap and with just 275 yards to go, just over half a lap, in his leather shoes and metal spikes he accelerated, took the lead and pulled away. The crowd screamed as he ran past them completing his final lap in 59 seconds.

When he crossed the line. Bannister said:

'My body must have exhausted its energy, but it still went on running just the same. The physical overdraft came only from greater willpower. This was the crucial moment when my legs were strong enough to carry me over the last few yards, as they could not have done in previous years.

'With 5 yards to go, the finishing line seemed almost to recede. Those last few seconds seemed an eternity. The faint line of the finishing tape stood ahead as a haven of peace after the struggle. The arms of the world were waiting to receive me only if I reached the tape without slackening my speed. If I faltered now, there would be no arms to hold me and the world would seem a cold, forbidding place. I leapt at the tape like a man taking his last desperate spring to save himself from a chasm that threatens to engulf him.

'Then my effort was over and I collapsed, almost unconscious, with an arm on either side of me. It was only then that real pain overtook me. It was as if all my limbs were caught in an ever-tightening vice. Blood surged from my muscles to my brain and seemed to fell me. I felt like an exploded flashbulb. Vision became black and white. I existed in the most passive physical state without being quite unconscious.'

Then there was a pause that filled the void with an indescribable tension and apprehension as the chief timekeeper, Harold Abrahams, handed a piece of paper to the announcer, Ross McWhirter. This was the historic announcement.

'Ladies and Gentlemen here is the result of the One Mile. First no 41 R. G. Bannister, Amateur Athletics Association and formerly of Exeter and Merton Colleges in a time which, subject to ratification, is a new track record, British native record, British all-comers record, European record, Commonwealth record and world record. The time was...three minutes...'

You couldn't hear the rest because of the noise of the crowd. I have goosebumps as I write this. He had done it; he had achieved the impossible.

So please take on board the message from one of the greatest athletes in history, take note and apply it to your own life. In a nutshell, rest and relaxation rejuvenates and is also essential to success.

So, is this the end of the story? No!

Within a month his time was beaten. Then, within three years, by the end of 1957, sixteen other runners also cracked the four-minute mile!

Was this due to a change in training methods or science behind muscle development? Absolutely not! It was a change in thinking that made all the difference. The challenge became possible which subsequently translated into belief. That word 'belief' is the most powerful of all words. Roger Bannister broke a mental barrier for the runners of the world. He believed! It was his attitude that influenced the result and got him over the line and delivered the time. If he believed it was impossible he would have never tried to break that barrier. Roger Bannister's belief changed the world that day and proves to this day that many of the barriers that hold us back exist only in our minds.

This quote captures this wonderful story in a few words . . .

'They did not know it was impossible so they did it.' ~ MARK TWAIN

PLUG IN TO YOUR LIFE FORCE

Let's now connect mind, body and spirit with that life energy, or life force referred to as *chi, qi* or *ki* I referenced in the green belt syllabus. In essence the belief is that every living thing has an energy that flows through it and outside of it, and, when unimpeded this is the fuel supply that provides life with zest and vitality. It is also a major concept in Eastern medicine as energy is said to travel around the body using special channels called meridians. In martial arts too, *chi* is 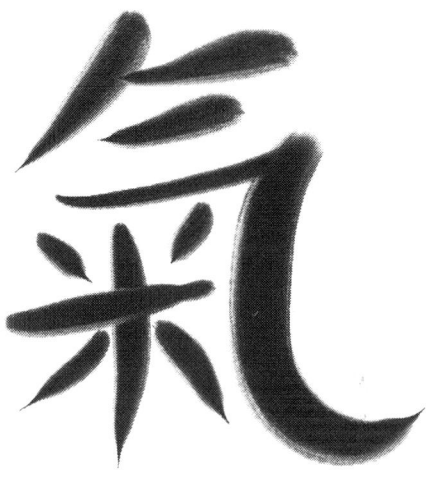 said to form spiritual strength. Along with the other ancient wisdoms and philosophies, the origin of *chi* has been traced as far back as 3,500 years.

It's believed that strong *chi* can have a positive effect on both mental and physical strength and offers protection against stressors from everyday life. Whereas a weak *chi* opens the door of negativity, impacting health and well-being.

Your *chi* is weakened by poor sleep and lack of nourishment, fresh air and clean water. Also, a lack of mental stimulation and social interaction. As with mindfulness, martial arts and yoga, there is much science available today to support these concepts and practices. It's as if much of humanity chose to ignore these ancient practices and knowledge, and only in the last few decades are we starting to appreciate exactly what these wisdoms can offer us all. We are starting to wake up and I hope this book contributes in some way to the awakening.

So how do you get your *chi* functioning? Where do we find that much-needed life energy? The answer lies in a word used repeatedly throughout this book – balance. Find that balance from evaluating everything we have discussed and applying it to your life. Don't forget to do it with moderation. Your life force will start to improve.

In summary, we need nourishing food and the right fluid intake for the body and stimulating mental nutrition for the mind. Connecting with others socially is vitally important for our mental health and then we must add movement to stimulate the body. Breathing clean fresh air, regular meditation and resting properly helps your body restore and rebalances your *chi*. Capture and unpack these last few paragraphs and overlay it onto your life. See what areas you are pleased with and which parts you might need help with.

So, to finish, think about this. *chi, qi* or *ki* is an Ancient Eastern concept that, in truth, can't be challenged! It's impossible to argue with it. Most of us just use different language such as: 'I'm on my A-game today', 'I feel great', 'I feel alive', 'I'm buzzing', 'I feel amazing today, full of energy and vitality'. Isn't this our *chi* showing its strength?

'A sound mind in a sound body, is a short, but full description of a happy state in this world.' ~ JOHN LOCKE

PURPLE BELT GRADING WARM-UP:

For the purple belt syllabus we dived deeper into wellness and identified what mind and body mastery is really all about. It's not having the mind of a genius and the body of an Olympic athlete. Mind and body mastery is showing awareness, listening, observing and responding to them both with care and attention. Please note that this is the way to living a black belt life.

We targeted a word, that in truth could become a philosophy; 'moderation', and how bringing a greater onus on balance into our lives could make a real difference.

We covered many aspects of how to develop mind and body mastery, all within your control, such as fitness, eating habits, nutrition and hydration, as well as the keystone of performance, the need for a healthy sleep pattern. Improving these essential life elements, many of which we take for granted, rewards you with greater heights of life experience.

Then we explored another ancient practice, yoga and the plethora of benefits it provides when practised regularly.

And finally, putting it all together has an amazing effect on our life force, that invisible energy referred to as *chi* or *ki*. This is mind and body mastery.

Once you have earned your purple belt, I want you to experience a new energy, another facet of the way to the black belt life. I want you to discover, understand and enjoy a quality of life in a more present and fulfilling way, really tuned in to your mind and, of course, your body. There is a Latin saying that goes, *'Mens sana in corore sano'.* This means 'a healthy mind is a healthy body'.

Good luck with your grading.

PURPLE BELT GRADING

1. *Mokuso* for two minutes. Sit quietly, close your eyes and gently focus on your breathing as learned as a green belt.
2. Centre yourself by reading 'The Man in the Glass'. The self-honesty you receive will fuel your spirit towards getting your purple belt.
3. Spend a short while reflecting on the syllabus.
4. Breakdown the elements of the syllabus and give yourself a performance score out of ten, with ten being perfection, against each part. This will help you find areas in need of attention. Try and target at least three areas to improve.
5. Can you add a brand-new feature to your life of wellness and well-being?
6. When do you feel at your best? When is your life energy at its peak? Start to evaluate how you feel in response to your lifestyle. Just assess it without judgement to see if there is any learning or development to be had.
7. Introduce stretching techniques into your daily life.
8. Work on becoming an observer of yourself. Listen carefully to your body. Make this a part of your life moving forward. Create a habit of checking-in and saying, 'Hi, how are you feeling?' Remember, mind and body mastery starts with knowing and understanding your body.
9. Check out your sleep pattern and relate it to your functioning and performance. Is there room for improvement?
10. Write in your book of life three key points you have taken away from this syllabus.

Congratulations!
You are now a purple belt.

'Purple is the last of the rainbow colours, so it means I will love and trust you for a long time.' ~ KIM TAEHYUNG

Please love and trust yourself first.

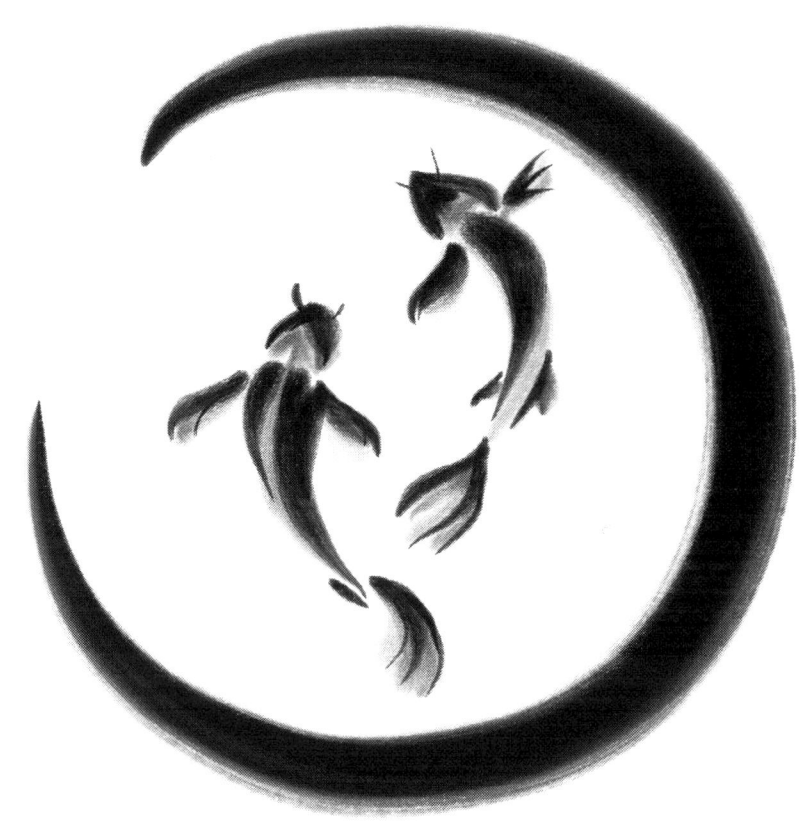

CHAPTER 7
BROWN BELT
Define your Purpose

'Life is never made unbearable by circumstances, but only by lack of meaning and purpose.' ~ VIKTOR FRANKL

We have been on a journey of transformation together, an expedition and exploration of the inner self. A unique trek that is personal to you and you alone. We have covered so much in the astonishing field of self-discovery and unlocked inner secrets and tools, drills and techniques to help you on the way.

Achieving brown belt status is about putting all the learning together to produce something that will power and stay with you for the rest of your life. When combined, the belts you have earned so far help you to determine the most significant and motivational aspects of your journey. You have now reached the part where the magic occurs. It's discovering the meaning and purpose to your life. This, my readers, is what drives us, what opens our eyes and gets us up in the morning. It's behind what we do and why we do it.

A large part of the brown belt syllabus focuses on reflection. Reflecting on what you have unearthed, learnt and how you have developed as a human being. Balancing and uniting the four quadrants of life; emotional, physical, spiritual and mental, in order to enjoy a life of well-being that's managed from the inside out.

'A black belt life' is very close now.

FIND YOUR *IKIGAI*

As a white belt you discovered the martial art of karate was developed in the Ryukyu Kingdom, an archipelago made up of 161 islands now named Okinawa and the birthplace of Gichin Funakoshi, the father of Shotokan karate and its twenty precepts. Now I want to transport you back to this extraordinary place. Yes, we are heading back to Okinawa, but this time to introduce you to its remarkable inhabitants and their unique lifestyle that has earned their island home its historic reputation as 'the land of the immortals'.

Okinawa has one of the highest concentration of centenarians, people who live past 100 years, than any other place on the planet and boasts some of the longest-lived people in history. Don't you think that is amazing? So, let's find out why.

They have a word that describes their secret. *Ikigai!*

Loosely translated, *ikigai*, means 'sense of purpose in life' or 'reason for being'. Iki means 'to live' and gai 'reason'. To the centenarians, *ikigai*, is an ethos, a way of life, a philosophy and a state of mind that allows you to live life to the fullest. This group of very special people have been the subject of much research to expose the secret of *ikigai*. Some experts who have studied the centenarians have said that knowing your sense of purpose is worth up to seven added years of life!

This book and the journey through it typifies the philosophy of this incredible group, the inside-out living approach to life. Behind this culture sits a mentality that true success is not measured by your wealth portfolio but by the joy and fulfilment you experience each and every day, and in this tiny part of the world, *ikigai* is the secret to experiencing just that. Astonishing facts relating to health and longevity are, by no coincidence, a reflection of the path to living a black belt life.

In essence, it all comes down to what we consume, what we do, who we connect with and, most importantly, what we think – our attitude to life. Sounds simple doesn't it? Well, we know full well it's not.

The true and full translation of *ikigai* is 'power necessary for one to live in this world, happiness to be alive, benefit, effectiveness'. The Japanese language is pretty ambiguous, so our English translation is, roughly speaking, 'purpose or meaning to live'. And I must stress the point it's *our* meaning and purpose of life and no one else's. Once again the message is it's about the self – it's about you.

I must drive home the message that the way of a black belt life is unique to each individual and will be interpreted and processed in your own special way. We are all different shapes, sizes, ages and minds. We are logical thinkers, creative thinkers and incentivised by a spectrum of different things. Therefore, you must use the tools as you see fit and find the secret to getting the best out of them. What I will say at this stage is 'reflect deep', as deep as you can, to find what works best for you and you will continue to discover more treasures within.

Let's now attempt to comprehend why Okinawa is 'the land of the immortals' and discover your *ikigai*.

Happiness and having fun are central to the lives of the inhabitants of the land of the immortals. Happiness is what fuels the fire of their lives. Happiness is infectious; surround yourself with like-minded, happy people and you will become infected with something good that could last a lifetime, as the Okinawans can vouch.

Neuroscience comes into play here in the form of mirror neurons, one of the most important neuroscientific discoveries in recent times and hugely significant in our role and ability to connect and socialise with others. Mirror neurons are brain cells that fire up when we observe actions performed by another person, mentally stimulating that feeling in ourselves. Smiling, for example, has been deemed to be neurologically contagious. When we smile or see someone else smile it stimulates positive neurological activity, which lifts our mood and reduces stress. Smiling boosts dopamine and raises our feeling of happiness. As I mentioned earlier, surrounding yourself with like-minded people, when you think about it, is the right thing to do. You feed off positivity, you feed off encouragement, you feed off upbeat people, you learn from them and begin the metamorphosis into becoming similar beings.

Let me remind you that the opposite can also occur. Our health and well-being choices can be influenced by our friends. It's not just peer pressure it's the brain picking up signals from the people around you that determines your behaviour. There is a significant chance that if many within our friendship circle have poor diets and are obese, we will edge towards this behaviour, too. For example, when we are with people who eat a lot, we tend to do the same and we are not always aware of this. There has been a great deal of interesting research on this phenomenon. The message here is be yourself and don't sway from what works for you when you have established your personal, well-balanced, well-disciplined wellness system.

The Okinawans genuinely feel good and fulfilled inside and have developed an inner harmony, which, through a ripple effect, influences the outside world they come in contact with. Yet again, this symbolises the learning gained on your own the journey from white to black. When you examine their lives they actually typify almost the perfect state of well-being.

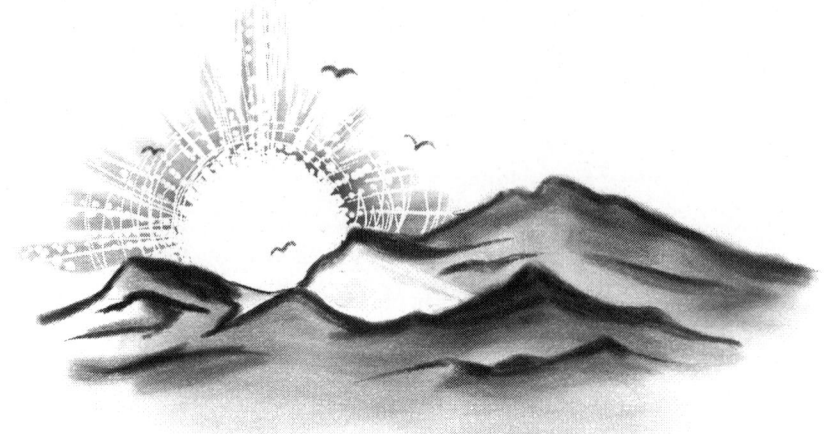

One of the Okinawan centenarian rituals is getting up early every day, usually when the sun rises, in order to obtain the fullness of what each day has to offer. They also spend time in touch with nature, spend time outdoors and bring outdoors indoors in the form of plants, pictures, paintings and prints of natural things. If you think about it, Japanese gardens are famous for their attention to detail.

They eat amazingly well, have a balanced diet, much of which is plant based and from the ground – fresh, never processed. They do things in moderation and keep under what the average calorie count is for men and women, but they do it consciously. They don't wait till they are full, bloated and exhausted to stop eating. They just stop.

And this is a crucial part of their superhuman well-being strategy – they move around a lot! That's it! Sorry if you were expecting something more profound. No, these guys will take the stairs not the escalator. They walk to their destination if they can. They exercise, practise yoga, Thai chi, Qi Gong (pronounced Chi Gong) or just stretch regularly.

They are always connecting with others, family and friends, living in harmony with them all. They are people-people, always sharing and enjoying others' company. These people also possess a conscious and meticulous attention to detail and that is the reason they show respect to everything they do and everyone they meet.

They have an innate quality of self-acceptance, something which is alien to many and is pivotal to finding peace and harmony in the world. Understanding and appreciating your strengths and weaknesses, areas that are in need of development and accepting these things is an amazingly liberating feeling and an incredible experience when it occurs. Then it becomes a part of who you are.

I worked with a female client who told me her story over the first two meetings. She really struggled just walking into the venue where we agreed to meet. She sat down opposite me with her self-esteem, confidence, her entire self-worth in shreds. She was timid, quiet, nervous and quivered when she spoke. Within a short while, tears were streaming down her face.

She had had such a traumatic upbringing and suffered a horrifying experience that no girl should endure in her early teens. This then resulted in eating disorders which still trouble her today, many years on.

I was totally immersed in her story as it unfolded. I was locked into it, I'm not sure I blinked as I was glued to her brief, but eloquent and articulate, account of her life to date. Alongside all this she had worked hard on her career, having many setbacks along the way, but relentlessly soldiering on and achieving incredible success. She is one of the most kind and caring people you could ever wish to meet, she is successful, married with a young family, with her whole life in front of her.

When she came to the end of this incredible synopsis of her life, I paused and reflected, before saying, 'Wherever do you get your strength from? You are so strong!'

She stared at me, silently, for what seemed like minutes, and then said, 'What! You think I'm strong?'

She went on to say that 'strong' was one word that's never been used by others to describe her and, most certainly, not by herself. At that moment she realised and recognised that one of her strengths was actually strength. She was strong, resilient, brave; she had something special about her, something to build on and be proud of.

From that moment on this amazing lady began her transformation. She found a way to accept that she had a gift, a gift of strength which instantaneously became her platform on which to build a new life. She is, for me, the perfect example of how your experience of the outside world can change if you can begin to observe, understand and accept the inner world. Paradoxically, accepting yourself releases yourself.

Celebrating who you are is pivotal to being able to live a life that focuses on self-development and self-growth, that black belt life. The Okinawan centenarian's philosophy is to live another day and learn something new. How beautiful is that?

When you put the Okinawan centenarians' way of life under a microscope you discover their magical key, it's staring right back at you.

They spend their time in the present moment, mindfulness is their secret, their magic. You can't be happy in the past, nor the future, you can only experience happiness in the present moment. They respect each moment and pay attention to it, and this is why they have a relentless attention to detail and quality. They are masters of the here and now, self-acceptance and self-awareness. This attitude symbolises so much of Japanese culture; they pay attention with intention to do things right and get things right. Attitude is reflected in a person's actions. Let's remind ourselves of the white belt philosophy – attitude is everything. What that means is that attitude is a way of life, not something that comes and goes. Attitude, nevertheless, is within our control.

Now let's revisit the key components discovered about the lifestyle of the inhabitants of the land of the immortals. They spend time outdoors and are in tune with nature. They have a well-balanced diet, eat wisely, and do not overeat. They spend time with family and friends. They move around, with lots of walking and natural body movements. They are masters of self-acceptance and demonstrate a mindfulness-based ideology; with a positive outlook and spiritual aspect to life. When you are at peace with yourself, comfortable in your own skin, you find the worrying stops and the freedom to express yourself starts. By the way, retirement is not a word in the Okinawan dictionary, they simply don't accept it. They just carry on with a purpose that transcends them, even when they become centenarians. In short, they purposefully live a black belt life.

But what is the key ingredient? What drives them each and every day, what gets them up in the morning? Do they have a secret extra component to add to a life of well-being?

Yes, of course they do. It's their *ikigai*, their singular, personal life purpose. The passion and vitality that brings meaning and value to life for this astonishing set of human beings. And this is your next test, to discover and acknowledge your *ikigai*. Your meaning, your *ikigai* is everything that brings joy to your life and if you can locate your *ikigai* this is the part that brings everything together. It makes it all worthwhile, and your journey changes as it becomes not only clearer and calmer but less daunting and less challenging. It's so much more exciting. This is living a black belt life in the pursuit of becoming the best you can be.

You all have an *ikigai*, for those of you who feel that you haven't, or it's been lost, I can tell you that it's buried along with those other treasures such as self-esteem, confidence, self-belief, joy, wisdom and clarity.

Your *ikigai* is unique to you. It can be simple and meaningful to you in a way it may not be to others, or it can be an outrageous, a life-changing ambition. It can be your philosophy. Remember, it's what gets you up in the morning, what opens your eyes every day.

Dan Buettner, an award-winning journalist, explored the lifestyle traits of centenarians and why the Okinawans have the highest life expectancy in the world. In a TED Talk, he cites the *ikigai* for one 102-year-old Okinawan karate master as being to continue teaching martial arts. The *ikigai* for a 101-year-old fisherman was catching fish for his family three times a week, whereas another 102-year-old Okinawan, this time a lady, stated that her *ikigai* is to hold her great-great-great-granddaughter. When Dan asked her what this felt like, she said, 'It's like leaping into heaven.' Two ladies separated by 101 years, isn't that just incredible.

Your *ikigai*, together with your curiosity, learning and self-discovery will strengthen that personal protection system against the outer world. Some people believe that having *ikigai* reduces anxiety because of the regular secretion of those happy hormones – serotonin, dopamine and endorphins. It makes you more resilient as you tough things out when you have a purpose to live, an *ikigai*. It helps to reduce the need to seek approval, why would you when you are at peace with your life? It's even been suggested through many scientific studies that *ikigai* is good for your heart, as people without it showed a higher mortality risk mostly due to cardiovascular disease. Basically, the findings were that people who believe their lives are worth living, live longer.

The Oshaki Study, cited in the online journal of the NIH National Library of Medicine, investigated the association between the sense of 'life worth living *(ikigai)*' and the cause-specific mortality risk. The study consisted of 43,391 adults being asked the question 'Do you have *ikigai* in your life?' The report continued to say that, over seven years, 3,048 of the subjects died. The risk of all-cause mortality was significantly higher amongst the subjects who did not find a sense of *ikigai* compared to ones that did. In this prospective study, subjects who did not find a sense of *ikigai* were associated with an increased risk of all-cause mortality. The increase in mortality risk was attributable to cardiovascular disease and external causes, but not cancer.

In another study by the Japan Collaborative Cohort (JACC), conducted from 1988 to 1990, a total of 30,155 Japanese men and 43,117 Japanese women aged between forty and seventy-nine completed a lifestyle questionnaire that included a question about *ikigai*. The findings concluded that a positive psychological factor such as *ikigai* is associated with longevity among Japanese people.

With your *ikigai* firmly in place, previously insurmountable challenges become small bumps in the road, and you will not experience emotional lows such as that life-threatening feeling you get when an aircraft suddenly drops altitude and turns your stomach inside out. Your emotional journey smooths out and the bandwidth between highs and lows becomes narrower and less dramatic. Dealing with adversity and trauma will always create pain but you are now stronger and more equipped to deal with it. It doesn't matter if you are a seamstress or a surgeon, an accountant or an astronaut, having a life purpose changes you. Our survival system doesn't know the difference between being faced by a rattlesnake or redundancy. Both are processed as threats, which trigger our fight or flight response, as covered in the yellow belt. Ikigai helps us through these situations and is our inner natural resistance to stress, working in the same vein as gratitude and love.

Throughout the book, we have focussed on the four parts of being; the quadrant of life. The *ikigai* glues them all together. For me, it manifests as your *chi* or *ki,* your life force, which, in turn, ignites that positive ripple effect of self-esteem, self-confidence, self-belief and self-improvement. An exponential spiral of growth, whereas self-pity, self-hate and being self-conscious will keep your *ikigai* deeply buried and difficult to find.

Your journey so far has been a roadmap for you to locate your *ikigai,* it has been referred to as more of a treasure map, due to the extent of the discovery, as I alluded to in the white belt syllabus. Please note, it's important to continue to use your own innermost vehicle to find it.

Remember, your life purpose doesn't have to be wealth related, it's so much deeper than that in terms of

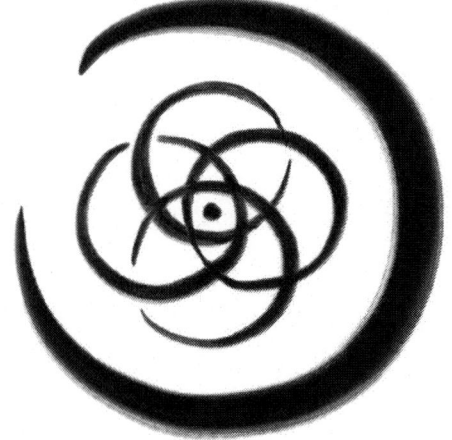

your rewards. It will manifest in lots of different and richer ways with the number one reward being happiness. If wealth, fame and fortune come along, so be it.

This is your toughest syllabus to date as it takes you close to your black belt. This exercise will help you discover and connect to your *ikigai*. As with all gradings this one requires you to commit fully to the process but, in addition, to search really deep in your self-reflection.

This will be the deepest dive you make to discover what gets you up and fires you up each day. This, my readers, is the part that accelerates your journey to sensei, being a black belt at whatever you do, whoever you are. This is the opportunity to put it all together. You just need to locate your *ikigai*.

According to neuropsychologist Ken Mogi, author of *The Little Book of Ikigai,* there are five parts to *ikigai*.

1. **Starting small**
2. **Releasing yourself**
3. **Harmony and sustainability**
4. **The joy of little things**
5. **Being in the here and now**

If you consider your journey through the grades you will have explored all these elements. Throughout this book, self-awareness and self-reflection are the fundamental keys. It's now time to reflect on what you have learnt and discovered.

1. **STARTING SMALL**
   As a white belt you had to take the first step through the metaphoric door and enter the dojo, the place of the way. It was a tiny step, but so courageous, too. A tiny step out of any comfort zone and into the unknown can deliver huge results. As a white belt we know nothing but to make that first move at the call of the instructor. We have then taken the first step on the path of the way to something very special. Remember that small steps can produce gigantic results.

2. **RELEASING YOURSELF**

   Through your journey from orange to red you built a belief structure that contains your value system and things in life you are most grateful for. You also took a deep dive into what your strengths are, what you like about yourself. By rediscovering and recognising these inner treasures you actually experience a shift towards greater confidence and empowerment, your self-esteem rises, and you start to release yourself from your fears and limitations. This is the start of breaking free, a psychological freedom which in turn creates a positive change in your perception of certain things. Things don't appear to be as challenging when you possess a secure belief structure and you're armed with your kitbag of life tools.

3. **HARMONY AND SUSTAINABILITY**

   During the yellow belt syllabus, we discovered the power of the mind and how it can be a gift or a curse. We discovered that we could find alignment and live in harmony with our values and beliefs, but also our limitations and areas we feel we could develop. We can use the power of the mind to our advantage creating a harmonious mindset that positively impacts others and is sustainable throughout our lives.

4. **THE JOY OF SMALL THINGS**

   You will have noticed that your attention to detail to the things that matter has grown. Small things that one would normally take for granted become important. As we transcended into the green belt we explored and discovered the many facets of mindfulness and gratefulness and how we can tune in to become more aware and appreciate things we previously took for granted. Moments that last for just seconds and arrive and disappear into the sea of life. These moments, these small things, are there for us to capture, pay attention to and enjoy. As a purple belt we checked into the physical side of life, again those things that we may take for granted such as what we consume and what we do and why we do it. Just taking time out to listen and observe from the inside out will reward you greatly in many ways.

5. **THE HERE AND NOW**

    This is the perfect way to describe mindfulness, which is underpinned by spending time in the present and cultivating the skills to nurture more of the precious moments in life. Being in the moment removes the past and future, and with it the regrets, guilt and anxiety and helps you to adopt a more positive mentality. It increases the sharpness of our experiences, and all our senses become more acute the more mindful we are. It's a magnificent way to learn that was never taught at school. Remember you can only be happy in the here and now.

So, according to Ken Mogi, these are the five parts to *ikigai*, the framework of that meaning and purpose which drives you each day. The synergy with the way of the black belt life is quite remarkable and, on reflection, when you take the results from the 'One Word' survey at the beginning of this book, it makes total sense.

During a client meeting I experienced a moment when a client I was coaching found his *ikigai*; his own meaning and purpose. He had been diagnosed with clinical depression and type 2 diabetes, within a month of each other, at the age of thirty-seven. This was devastating for him. He felt his world had ended, as his doctor and the NHS had officially diagnosed his depression through a series of examinations.

It then occurred to him that he had been depressed for many years, which compounded the realisation. He was in a chronic state of stress; an everlasting flux of fight or flight. At this time, he felt alone and helpless, he broke down as he grasped the enormity of what he had just been told.

He called me and asked me to work with him. He spoke to me while staring at a packet of antidepressants he had been prescribed and just picked up from the chemist. He said to me, 'I want to work with you as I know you're a winner, you never give up. And that's what I need, I need to work with someone for whom failure isn't on the radar.'

His coaching journey was a tough one, to say the least, but it was also an astonishing one. Working together, we uncovered his goals whereby it became clear he wanted to reverse both illnesses. But in his mind, progress had to be proven clinically by taking the same tests that resulted in the prognosis.

This was a gargantuan challenge but a fantastically inspirational one. We went for it and proceeded to plot out his journey. To even get somewhere close we realised that there needed to be huge changes to his lifestyle. His eating habits, his nutrition, fitness, exercise planning, how he rests and recovers and more. He was advised to lose a considerable amount of weight and needed to take immediate action. To accomplish this, he had to find an inner belief and change in mindset.

Being a hardworking and successful business owner with a committed hands-on approach to work he understood the need to incorporate all these changes into his twenty-four-hour day including his ten-to-twelve-hour working days.

Think about it. It's tough enough for some people to give up smoking, cut down on their chocolate consumption or introduce a little more exercise in their lives. It's a challenge for sure, and as we have covered along the way, creating new habits is most certainly not easy.

Now, this guy had to make a number of drastic lifestyle changes and to accomplish them he needed mental strength, a genuine determination and an attitude of discipline, commitment and perseverance. He needed that ultra-strong mental platform to make these changes.

We set out on our journey together using the six pillars of the way as our go-to to ensure we stayed on track and became accountable. Piece by piece, he started to turn things around. He worked so incredibly hard incorporating the changes he had to make and applying the necessary discipline when and where needed.

If you used this book as a measure of his progress, he became an orange belt very quickly, then red, by building a belief structure and defining some inspirational goals. He committed to building his mental core strength to help strengthen his confidence, self-esteem and self-belief. Each week we added more mental reps to his routine and new tools into his life that continued to shore up his motivation, confidence and self-worth. He went through his belts of life with relentless determination.

The truth is that along the way he had what we described as 'wobbles' whereby temptation would ease him away from his strict lifestyle changes. He would get incredibly frustrated when he succumbed to temptation. This resulted in some regret, guilt and taking little steps backwards.

We had clear goals, we had a belief structure in place, we had a solid plan and process set up. And he was doing brilliantly. But what was missing? His true meaning and purpose, his *ikigai*. We both realised that, although it was hidden, it wasn't far away. It's been said that you have to go through the darkness to find the light switch, and we were close to finding it.

What happened next? We were in the middle of a session together and we were unpacking the quite remarkable prospect of clinically reversing both type 2 diabetes and his diagnosed major depression.

I mentioned to him that, alongside this book, I intended to produce accompanying podcasts about living the black belt way and that his story could be a message of encouragement to many people out there. That was it, the light came on, he'd found it. His face changed, his body relaxed and, with a smile, he said, 'Bring it on.' He found his *ikigai*. It was to help others suffering with similar conditions.

I have to mention that in less than six months I received a text from him saying he had officially and clinically reversed his depression. It read, 'one down and one to go'. I cannot tell you how that made me feel. I was blown away.

He went on to say he had made it known to the NHS nurse that he had not received any follow-up after being diagnosed with depression and hadn't taken one of the antidepressants she had prescribed to him. She asked, 'Why not?'

He responded, 'You didn't call back, and I found a coach instead who has changed my life.'

It was a touching moment for me reading that, it meant everything. I'm constantly inspired and driven by clients such as this young man and how he faced up to adversity. I reminded him that it was not me who changed his life, it was all down to him.

You will see I use the term 'deep dive' a lot and this guy has, and is, still diving deep into his soul, his inner self, to find those hidden treasures and reserves of wisdom and strength to change his and others' lives.

I was mulling over whether to include this story, but in October, 2021, I received another text from him. 'Blood results are in...great call with diabetes consultant today. I am where I need to be. Got to maintain for three months. I said to her, don't worry I'll smash it.'

He went on to say that the consultant was majorly impressed as it was rare that people reverse type 2 that quickly.

Moving forwards to the morning of 2nd February, 2022 I received this text: 'Guess what?'

I replied with an emoji of me praying.

'I'm off the meds'.

It was a moment of sheer joy. It's difficult to describe how I felt, let alone my client. And now he wants to share his story to inspire others.

As a white belt I explained that the answers are all within us. It's our inner world that will provide them, not the outer world. People constantly look outwards to move forward in their lives or seek peace and happiness outside. We forget to look the other way and shine that torch of life back at us.

Michael Neill, in his book *Supercoach,* refers to an ancient Sioux legend:

In ancient times the creator wanted to hide something away from humans until they were ready to use it. He gathered together all the other creatures of creation to ask them for their advice.

The eagle said, 'Give it to me and I will put it on top of the highest mountain in all the land.'

The creator said, 'No, one day they will conquer the mountain and find it.'

The salmon said, 'Leave it with me and I will hide it at the bottom of the ocean.'

But the creator said, 'No, humans are explorers at heart and one day they will go there too.'

The buffalo said, 'I will take it and bury it in the heart of the great plains.'

The creator said, 'No, one day the skin of the earth will be ripped open and they will find it there.'

The creatures of creation were stumped. But then an old blind mole spoke up. 'Why don't you put it inside them, that's the last place they will look.'

The creator said, 'It is done.'

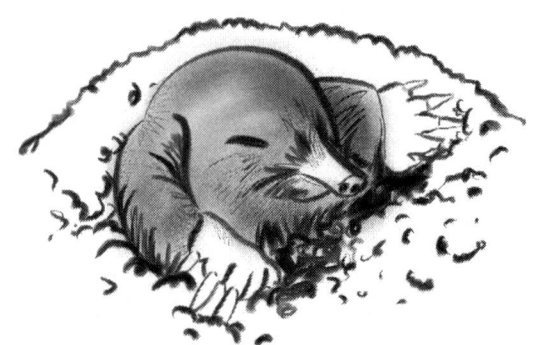

To end this chapter, I'd like to share with you the story of what happened when I momentarily lost sight of my own *ikigai*, and a second 'angel' entered my life.

A number of years ago, close to fifteen I believe, a feeling of demotivation entered into my life. It sort of crept up on me over a period of time and then it became clear that something was not right with the emotional side of my well-being. I couldn't identify the problem and I was confused. I didn't know if it was, perhaps, an episode of depression manifesting itself in a way I had never before experienced.

It felt like someone had knocked the edges off my zest and vitality for life. The brightness to my life seemed to have faded. I felt a sadness had appeared and I started to carry something that was familiar to me; a weight in my chest. It wasn't dramatic and nothing like on the level that the Amazing Fred suffered, but it was there nonetheless. This continued for some time, and it became a part of who I was; it felt normal.

Then I had a chance meeting with a guy at my gym.

I was in the crowded changing room, getting changed into my karate gi for training and a man I did not recognise enquired, quite loudly, above the chatter, 'Are you Phil Toogood?' I answered yes, and he made his way over to me.

He then told the story of when he had played cricket against me many years before. I was a pretty aggressive fast bowler, so I asked him about that day with a feeling of anticipation. He said that I bowled particularly aggressively which had upset a few of his teammates but, interestingly, not him. He had been impressed by my competitive spirit and attitude and always remembered it. My memory relating to games played, runs scored, and wickets I took was, and is, very sketchy. But this particular game had stayed in this gentleman's memory. That was our first brief meeting and I went to train in the dojo.

At that time, I used to take a sauna after karate training to stretch my muscles and relax. A couple of weeks later, I opened the door of the sauna and this same guy was sitting in there on his own. We started a conversation which led to me unpacking some of the emotional challenges I was experiencing at the time. I have no idea why, but I did and in some detail, too. He also shared with me some of his own challenges he had battled with. We hit it off and it was good to talk about what I was feeling. It just felt right. After thirty minutes or so we parted company.

Two weeks later, I was in the sauna again, this time on my own, and this guy entered. He said hello, and then went on to say this. 'I've been thinking a great deal about our conversation the last time we met and I think I know what your problem is.

'Phil, you mentioned you had recently retired from cricket. Now, think about it. For nearly thirty years you have been not just competing in this sport, but excelling in it as a player, captain, coach, chairman... Nearly every week your name has appeared in the local press. Week in, week out, you would perform with your bowling and batting, and you played in, and captained, championship-winning sides. Your weekends during all this time were about competing in a sport you love, receiving accolades, pats on the back and newspaper headlines.

'You spent three decades as part of team and a club. You were a team player and loved the changing room environment being with great friends but also the training, the planning, the winning and the celebrating...

'And Phil, now it's all gone! All of it has stopped! This was a massive and magnificent part of your life and it is no more. No more changing room, no more headlines, no more five-wicket hauls when bowling, centuries when batting or diving catches when fielding...no more pats on the back and being part of a team.

'This is exactly, and I mean *exactly*, why you are suffering.'

He was right, I'd lost my *ikigai*.

In that moment, everything changed. He had discovered the problem and administered the antidote so eloquently. He helped me to understand my problem and then absorb it into my system. It was simply remarkable. I was then able to reframe my mindset and set new challenges within my life including the world of karate.

But that's not the end of the story. My readers, the goosebumps have appeared.

I never saw this gentleman ever again. Ever!

He came into my life just three times, once in a busy changing room and twice in an empty sauna, but within those three brief meetings he healed me of the pain and suffering I was experiencing and carrying at that precise time. He helped me to rediscover my *ikigai*.

I believe this person was, indeed, an angel.

BROWN BELT GRADING WARM-UP:

The test to become a brown belt is to put together all the learning gained so far from white to purple. I liken it to building a spiritual machine that delivers the life skills and tools most of us seek. A re-engineering project to deliver a new version of ourselves through our learning. So, what is the fuel that drives this machine, this amazing life system we are building? It's our true meaning and purpose. The thing that gets us out of bed each morning.

We visited the island where karate originated from and made friends with some incredible people from the land of the immortals, the Okinawan centenarians who live longer on average than anyone, anywhere on the planet. We explored the reasons behind this incredible statistic and walked away with some answers and understanding relating to their uniquely special code to living. We found the password to allow us to enter into the mainframe of their philosophy of living a happy, peaceful and fulfilling life. The password is *ikigai*.

Ikigai stitches together all the learning, it drives your motivation to keep moving forward. Keeping with the message that flows through this book like the purest, crystal-clear stream, your *ikigai* is within you, buried along with the abundance of other wonders you had locked away.

By finding your *ikigai* and becoming a brown belt you are ready to take the next step, that final, extraordinary and life-changing step to the home of the black belt.

Here's your brown belt grading.

Good luck to you all.

BROWN BELT GRADING

1. Revisit all gradings so far and journal any key points you gained but also any you might have missed.

2. Is your value system still intact? Is it complete or can you add to it? Remember you can add values to your system when you need to change for the better or possibly alter your direction slightly. This works, as long as you are loyal to the value(s) you have added.

3. Ask yourself, 'What am I really good at?' It can be anything. Revisit past successes and achievements. What are your strengths? Where does your potential lie and how can you realise it?

4. Are you making a difference somewhere? If so, where? If not, how could you give back to society? What would you teach if you could?

5. What is your passion(s) in life? What do you love doing? Remember that saying, love what you do or do what you love. Is there something inside your working environment or outside of it. Write it down.

6. What areas of self-development would like to explore?

7. Do you have a better understanding and control of your emotions? Are you now including mindfulness into your life, if so how?

8. How do you see the world, do you have a positive outlook?

9. What is your personal well-being structure? Break it down and note all the changes you have made.

10. How do you want to be remembered? How do you want to be described by others? What is your legacy?

11. Produce a word or make up a sentence that describes clearly your *ikigai*. My official version is: 'To learn and develop, to share and transform'. My spiritual version is: 'To feel alive'.

You should now be able to answer the question: WHAT IS YOUR *IKIGAI*?

Congratulations!
You have become a brown belt.

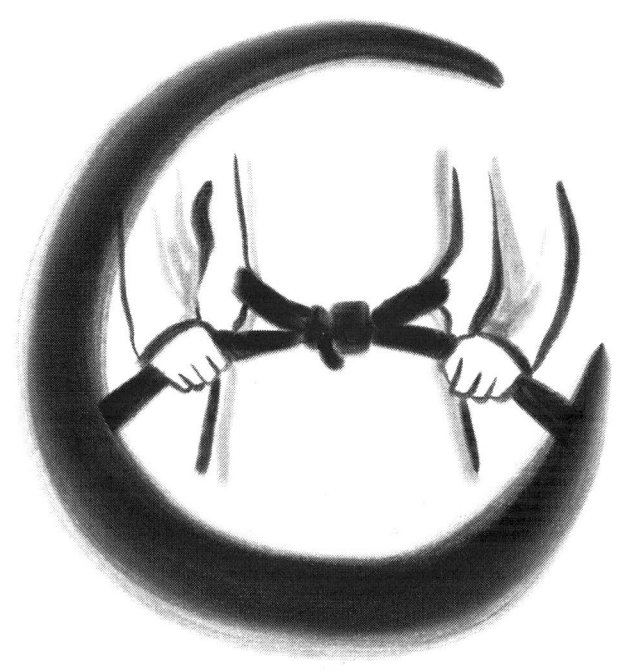

CHAPTER 8
BLACK BELT
Sensei

'To follow the path, look to the master, follow the master, walk with the master, see through the master, become the master.' ~
ZEN PROVERB

This is it; you are here. This is the black belt syllabus; designed to deliver the respected status of sensei along with that magical final belt. This chapter will take you to another level. It will continue to challenge you but with a change in dynamic and direction.

You have been on such an amazing journey across the dojo of life and are approaching that magical place where the elite hang out. This is a very special place indeed. It's somewhere full of feelings, emotions and accomplishments, supported by continuous learning on another level to what you've experienced along the way.

It's quite an extraordinary space to stand in. There is an outer body presence and energy that comes with the territory. The people who operate in that far right place are living proof that the six pillars of the way undoubtedly work when you apply them to a goal, especially a really challenging goal.

Karate students train for years to get a shot at a black belt but going from brown to black is an entirely new experience. It's about revisiting everything that has been discovered and learned and then honing and polishing each move and striving for perfection while demonstrating an attitude rich in spirit, heart and resilience.

We work tirelessly to harness the skills, energy and power we have discovered, developed, refined and then stockpiled to unleash in the right place at the right time to achieve maximum results. Can we do the same in life? Yes, we can.

All that work, all that dedication to unlock the hidden potential within, discovering things about yourself you never knew existed. Facing and embracing your fears and limitations, understanding what makes you tick and how that can be translated into performance, culminating in living a happier, rewarding and more fulfilling life.

The grading exam for black belt is very different to the others. Yours will be different, too. We will go back to basics but also unpack any 'aha' moments and breakthroughs along the way that have created a shift in your thinking, actions and direction. And then we will review some of the tools that are now in your kitbag of life.

Watching other students transition from a white belt to a black belt is one of the most inspirational things I have ever witnessed. It literally takes years of grit, determination, resilience and resolve to get there. It feels incredible to be a part of other people's life journeys and their success brings many different types of reward. The same can be applied to my coaching practice outside the dojo and was also the inspiration behind writing this book.

An incredible ripple effect takes place whereby so many other people benefit from one person's growth. It can be a partner, parent, friend, relative, student, work colleague, your child or teammate. All these people profit from your growth.

As we are getting close to that moment, I want you to really focus your attention on every word. I want this day to be a very special event for you. I want it to be a big day in your life, as it was for me.

I would like to share with you what happened to me on my big day. This is the story of my grading, the most intensely testing examination of my life, the day that all those years of training culminated in; this one day, one hour and for me it was one shot! I had prepared mentally and physically for this one time. I never included in my vision, planning or thought process anything other than this one event. I treated that one day as all or nothing.

It took place at a neutral venue. Black belt exams are never held at your club. Yet another example of taking you outside of your comfort zone. It was in Reading, which was a good two-hour drive for me. I had prepared as best I could, I had given everything and more in the lead-up and intentionally taken off the last two training sessions to rest and avoid injury.

I booked a hotel in Reading and drove down the night before, again to avoid any issues or potential stressors on the morning of my exam. I'm generally happy in my own company so I knew I wasn't going to sit and stress about the next day. I checked into my room, had dinner in the restaurant then headed back for an early night. All good so far and I woke up on the day of the grading feeling great, if a little tense.

However, when walking to my car in the hotel car park I slightly missed my footing stepping off a kerb and tweaked my knee. It resulted in a short, sharp pain I'd never experienced in all my years of playing sport. I couldn't believe it. Maybe I was more tense and tight than I realised? Then I changed my mindset and took control of the situation. I thought: *Stop whinging! Just give your knee a good rub, take some paracetamol and get on with it.* This was an example of the mental chatter that occurs when we are challenged.

I arrived at the venue, which was a modern sports centre. I could see what seemed like hundreds of people in white gis, heading towards the building. After a while, I realised I hadn't spotted anyone that was even close to my age. Everyone was a lot younger than me.

On grading day, everyone is expected to participate in a rigorous training session that lasts for one and a half hours before the grading commences. It's like a more intense version of a grading warm-up than you have ever experienced before. The training is delivered by one of the senseis from the examining team for the black belt grading. These guys are like gods in the world of karate.

There were about 100 or so in the training session. I did the session, putting 100% into every move, while being watched and instructed by the senseis, and in truth, backing off just a little to conserve my energy when they were focussed on another student. What happened to the sharp pain in my knee? It disappeared. Did I just mentally disregard it? Dismiss it as negative interference? I never felt it again!

My sensei, Peter, was watching from the gallery above and spotted that one of the moves in my *kata* was wrong. The moves in a *kata* range between twenty and sixty-five depending on the complexity. I must have been performing this particular move incorrectly for years and because it was so slight it had never been picked up by any of the senseis I had trained under. I now understand why; my sensei was looking down on me from up in the gallery and being in an elevated position it made the mistake clear to see. At ground level, it was almost impossible to spot. Can you believe that? On the day of my exam, I was told it was a wrong move and I would fail if I didn't correct it!

My sensei shouted down to explain what I was doing wrong. My heart started to pump, I began to hyperventilate; my emotions were all over the place and then panic set in. I now had to think about a new move on the day of my grading after spending years of practice honing and polishing this particular series of moves until they were lodged deep into my subconscious so I could execute them automatically to the highest possible standard. I had developed a perfect mind and muscle memory that now needed to be changed in one hour! It felt like an impossible task to create and embed a neural map for this new move in so short a time, so I was going to have to rely on my conscious state and short-term memory.

Suddenly, I was experiencing fight or flight. My PFC was shutting down as I went into panic mode (which we learnt about in the yellow belt syllabus). Then, I started to combat my panic, I guess unknowingly I deployed the samurai to fight off the fear of failure, but what else did I do? I found a quiet place to rehearse the new move and initiated *Mokuso*. I shut my eyes and focussed on my breath which brought me back to a state of in the moment calmness. I was back in the place I needed to be to succeed. The here and now.

I knew I had to take back control of the situation. I had no time to be angry, upset or emotional, I needed to respond, and respond well, to achieve the outcome I wanted. It was the perfect example of E+R=O. The 'O' outcome needed was me mastering this move, and quickly, therefore my 'R' had to be right.

Then the event began; there was no more time. This was what everyone had trained for, this day, this grading. No other grading had been, or would be, as significant as this one.

The atmosphere in the room was electric, there was a buzz of excitement mixed with an air of nervousness and anticipation, a tension like I had never experienced.

Suddenly, there was complete silence – it was as if 100 people stopped breathing. You could sense something; you could feel the senseis were on their way to the dojo. As they entered there was a discharge of noise generated from the thick white material of sixty or so gis as everyone stood in unison and bowed to the senseis. The atmosphere intensified and nerves increased to an almost unbearable level.

During the grading, the senseis are positioned at the end of a large mat on which the exam takes place, sitting down behind a table, and from there they announce their instructions in a loud but emotionless voice. They are delivered as orders, and you are expected to respond with perfection. The grading event begins with the youngest first and everyone else sits around the outside of the mat waiting to be called up to demonstrate their skills.

I sat at the edge of the mat for nearly three hours waiting to be called. I was the oldest grading, so I had to wait until last. I went through every emotion you can imagine while sitting there.

After the first hour of watching the younger students, I started to get cramp. You can't get up to stretch or move around as you are in a seated position on the floor and cannot disturb what is happening on the mat.

You just have to wait and deal with the mental and physical challenges as they arrive. The cramp got worse, and I was annoying the people around me with my constant fidgeting.

My mental guard dropped, my samurai took a break, and I let the mind trash sneak into my headspace to sabotage me. *What are you doing here? Why do you need to prove anything to anyone?* (The actual language in my head was a lot worse than that I must admit.) *Why do I need to keep challenging myself? Is it my ego?*

Then the inner enemy came out in force increasing its power. *Why not get up, bow to the floor and walk straight out the door. You don't need this. Leave now!*

What was going on in my head? I took a virtual step outside my experience and checked in to take a look. I almost laughed at my destructive thoughts. So, I captured those thoughts and dealt with them. I destroyed them using all the weaponry I had gained along my journey from the moment I walked into the dojo wearing a pair of blue tracksuit bottoms. I was determined to prove I could live a black belt life.

This is what happened next…

Swiftly, the thoughts and feelings started to fade away and were replaced with positive mantras. *Do you know what, I've nothing to lose? I have worked hard and prepared brilliantly, so what is my problem? I'm going to smash this out of the park, and I pity anyone who gets in my way.* Within a few seconds I had got out of the way of myself. It was a perfect example of p=P-I from the orange belt syllabus. I had freed me from myself, my thinking and my inner adversary. It was an amazing transformation.

It was like someone had flicked the switch to 'on', started the engine and I was going through an emotional set of gears, and then another to 'turbo'. I suddenly felt only excitement, self-belief and confidence. Then something quite extraordinary happened. This incredible feeling of quietness and calmness took over but also came with a laser-like focus that you dream about on the journey from white belt to where I was sitting. I was now in a special and sacred place, a zone of peak performance; I had the perfect neurochemistry going on, I had found the sweet spot in my brain and my thinking. I had just the right amount of stress, the positive kind that helps focus attention.

This peak level state is also known as Yerkes-Dodson law. It was discovered by scientists Robert Yerkes and John Dodson in 1908 that performance was poor with low levels of stress. They found that the sweet spot of performance occurred at reasonably elevated levels of stress and then tapered off at high levels. This phenomenon is referred to as the inverted U.

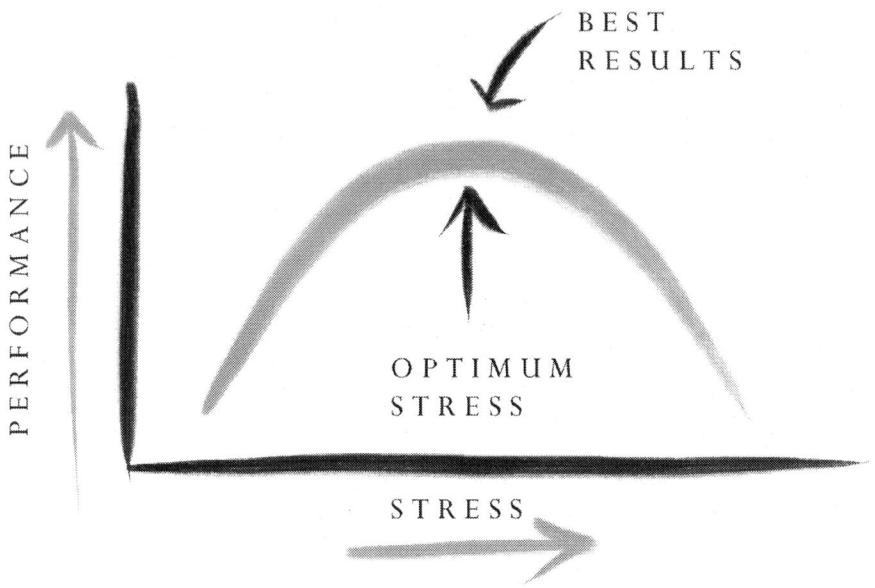

I was now in this amazing place with what felt like my mind, body and spirit in harmony. In truth, it felt like an out-of-body experience. I was in the moment, there was no past, no future, no cramp, no mental chatter and no expectation. I was in the here and now. It was an incredible place to be.

My name was eventually called out and I was up and out like a shot, positioned on the mat and ready to perform. Straight into the first move with the loudest 'kiai' I had ever done (this is a Japanese term used in karate for shouting when performing an attacking move).

You have probably seen when martial artists attack someone or break boards they scream throughout the action. There are many reasons for this. Some say it's a battle cry or used to startle an opponent but there is also some physiology supporting this phenomenon. Shouting helps you bring 100% focus to the move and outcome. Exhaling helps tighten the core which is where our power is stored as we covered as an orange and purple belt. Tightening the core also protects us from getting injured when taking a hit around the stomach area. A *'kiai'* shouldn't come from the throat it should come from the diaphragm.

I got through the first part of the exam completing my *kihon,* a series of basic moves, punches, kicks and combinations that must be performed to perfection. I left nothing out – I gave everything and then a bit more, every ounce of energy, too much in fact. I didn't hold back. It was the wrong strategy. The occasion and my attitude got the better of me and I'd forgotten what my instructor had said to me many months before about my karate. He said, 'You always give 100% to everything, in fact you try to give more and that's why you lose form and get injured. Rein it back, just a few percent and that will help you with your form, your technique, your balance and decision-making particularly when fighting.' My karate changed for the better from that moment.

This advice is something to reflect on in life and work towards. Give 100% commitment but allow yourself a slight cushion to help maintain focus, energy and clarity, allowing creativity, confidence and growth. It stops the wobble effect. This occurs when you are so tense you shake. We all experience the 'wobble effect' from time to time and backing off helps us press pause.

But within the intensity of this moment, I had forgotten to rein it in, and I was now hyperventilating again but with greater intensity at the edge of the mat holding up the three other guys going for their black belts alongside me. The senseis had to wait as I couldn't control my breath. I thought I might pass out. I remained in the correct position and posture to respond to their next instruction, which was a specific *kata* for the black belt grading. This was the *kata* I had engineered a wrong move into over the years.

Once I had regained control of my breathing which seemed to take a lifetime, the senseis screamed out the name of the *kata* and I had to explode into action and deliver forty-two moves to perfection – full power, perfect timing and with a spirit and attitude that surpassed anything I had done before. I plunged deep inside myself and found the resource from somewhere, and I nailed it. It was strange that when I got to that specific move, the one my sensei had noticed was wrong, I was facing him watching in the crowd. I delivered the move with precision and saw him nod.

By the time the *kata* finished my energy was all but spent. I was then paired up with another contender to demonstrate various attacks, combinations and defensive moves while under perfect control so as not to injure your opponent. This is your opportunity to show off all the years of training and the skills you have gained.

My opponent obviously had forgotten the control element of this discipline as he cracked me in the eye with a punch and kicked me in the midriff, subsequently flooring me. In this part of the grading exam there should be no full contact whatsoever only a touch of the gi to demonstrate perfect control.

A medic had to be called to assess me. I was struggling to see out of one eye for a while. I was cleared to continue, and we faced each other again. But this time it was full-on *kumite,* martial arts freestyle fighting, with a referee.

The previous blows I took from my opponent put me in an even higher state of flow, it took me back into the zone, that zone of peak performance. It was an incredible feeling, like a dream playing out, it was depersonalisation. I had no nerves anymore; I could have been alone with this guy although there were over 100 people watching in this small arena. We stood about ten feet apart when the referee yelled *'hajime'* which is Japanese for begin.

I had been practising a move for months in the dojo, outside the dojo, in my mind in the bath, in the shower… It was a move that wasn't taught as part of the syllabus, but I had perfected it. I must have practised this over a thousand times. There is a quote from an unknown source that says, *'Don't practise until you get it right. Practise until you can't get it wrong.'* This is exactly what I did with this technique.

This was a move that I owned. It was mine. It was a move that never failed to land a blow on my opponent even when their defences were up and ready. If delivered without control it was a guaranteed knockout blow that could cause some serious damage.

I changed my stance, then changed back again and then delivered this spinning blow to the side of my opponent's head covering the distance between us in a split second. I delivered it with complete control with the loudest *'kiai'* I could muster. I hit the guy before he even moved.

I heard the instructor, a former National, European and World Champion and the toughest sensei I had ever trained with as he was renowned for screaming at you if you didn't perform to his high standards, loudly shout, 'That was fantastic!' It was unheard of in a grading scenario, that an instructor would comment during any discipline. I will never forget that moment.

My neurochemistry must have reached the absolute optimum state. I had trained for years for this moment. I had prepared leaving no stone unturned. Bruce Lee said, *'I fear not the man who has practised 10,000 kicks once, but I fear the man who has practised one kick 10,000 times.'* I had endured all the mental, physical and emotional challenges, but my faith remained present along the way. I had reached the physical peak required but had to address my state of mind while sitting watching the people before me carry out their gradings. I proved you can flip negative thinking into a positive mindset in just a few minutes, even seconds.

When I look back, I can appreciate that I was in the perfect state of flow as highlighted in the yellow belt syllabus. This optimal experience was exactly how Mihaly Csikszentmihalyi described it. A state of being when people are so involved in an activity that nothing else seems to matter. And the concentration is so intense there is nothing left over to focus on problems or anything else. I truly believe that I also enter a sense of flow when I am coaching people.

I went on to destroy my much younger opponent, bringing with it many accolades from the edge of the mat and spectators in the gallery as I walked off. I looked across at my sensei and he smiled and gave me a soft and modest silent applause. I felt incredible. That is the only way to describe it. I was 100% spent but felt superhuman. I had switched my brain and my physiology into optimum performance mode!

If you made it through the three disciplines of *kihon, kata* and *kumite* then you were selected to deliver another *kata* but different to the last. They select one out of seven potential *katas,* so you have to know them all virtually blindfolded. No one knows until they are on the mat in the prepared position which *kata* they are going to call. Then the sensei thunders out the kata of their choice. The one they chose for me was a twenty-three-move *kata.* I nailed that, too.

You don't know if you've achieved black belt until all the grading students sit down at the end. Out of around sixty of us, just a handful of people passed. Being one of the last to grade I had to wait while the senseis went through each person and delivered a pass or a failure. You failed even if you passed three out of four disciplines.

I sat there and my villainous, doubtful mind kicked off again. *Had I done enough?* I was exhausted, suffering with physical and mental fatigue, so my thinking was leading me to get on that negative train of thought.

Eventually, my name was called and then those words I will never forget 'Pass *Shodan*'. That meant I'd now become a black belt. The goosebumps are appearing as I write this.

That was one of the most challenging things I have ever faced. I journeyed from white to black belt and became the first in the club to do so with no failures in any of my gradings. I was by far the oldest too, apart from my sensei. My daughter, Ellie, was to replicate this journey a few years later.

Why was this journey life-changing for me?

Because I spent almost the entire adventure outside of my comfort zone and although it's bit of a cliché, it was a true and honest journey of self-discovery. I discovered things about myself that I never knew existed and, from the moment the sensei announced I had become a black belt, it felt like I had become Superman. Everything changed, my self-esteem, my self-confidence and I gained a belief that I could take on almost anything. I experienced what it felt like to have a presence.

And this is my message to all my readers. A journey of transition leading to transformation can be achieved without entering the dojo. You do not need to find inner peace and fulfilment high up a mountain, on the jetty of a stunning lake, or watching the sun set on a remote beach on an island in the Indian Ocean. Of course, these are beautiful experiences, but the answers and inspiration are not at the end of the jetty, or on a beach or up the mountain. They are all within you, in your own private chamber of secrets.

EMOTIONAL INTELLIGENCE

When I look back at my karate journey I try and pinpoint certain circumstances that provided me with a shift of confidence, something that changed the way I felt, the way I thought and the way I behaved.

I asked myself these questions. What drives everything we do? Where does motivation and elite performance come from? Where does it start and where does it finish? How do we access it when it's needed most?

It always comes back to the power of the mind.

Appreciating some of the science and human evolution behind how we think and operate, will underpin your success as a person, whatever success looks like for you. And the more you understand, the more skilful you become at managing and controlling your emotions. It's called Emotional Intelligence (EI) or Emotional Quotient (EQ).

We have looked at how some people have presence, they hold themselves upright and have an air of calm confidence, along with an almost unfathomable combination of humility with a little fear attached. So, what separates them from the rest? Emotional Intelligence.

EI is exactly what is says; being intelligent about your emotions! The master of EI, the incredible Dr Daniel Goleman, author and psychologist,

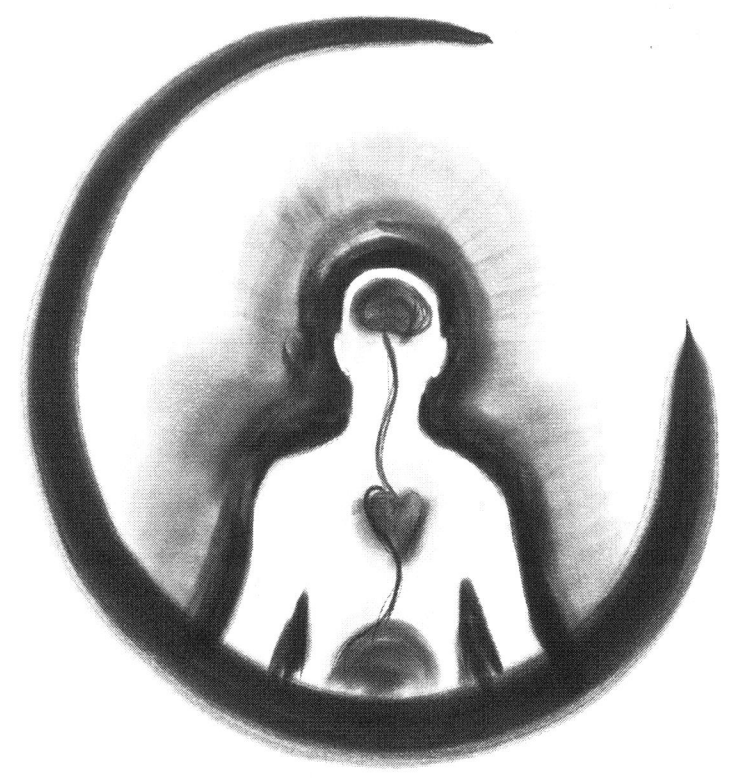

describes it as *'a person's ability to manage their feelings so that those feelings are expressed appropriately and effectively'.*

Now, please reflect on this for a moment...

Along your journey from white to black belt we specifically targeted the sense of self in many ways to establish first truth, and then growth. Developing greater self-awareness has been key throughout. In addition, you are so much more in tune with your core values and your inner strengths, and that raises your levels of self-confidence and, of course, most important of all, self-belief. These elements make up your belief structure your fortress. I must add that, as with some permanent structures, they still need to be maintained, repaired and strengthened. The important thing is that the structure is in place so that it can be continuously improved, extended, expanded and built upon.

You have also learned how, when and why our inbuilt fight or flight survival system is deployed and how we can keep it in a heightened state through negative and, sometimes, catastrophic thinking patterns that translate into stress and anxiety or depression. By becoming the observer as well as the thinker, you can be your own eyewitness to your emotional manifestations. You have learned to recognise them and acknowledge how they incarnate and why you are experiencing them. It's like joining the dots of the entire experience from the origin of the event to the emotional outcome. This breakthrough in conscious awareness enables you to reduce the power and energy of emotional pain and amplify feelings of joy, excitement and happiness. Gaining command and control of your emotions develops into a game changer. Self-reflection and self-acceptance are the launch pad of EI and these life-changing skills fall under the spiritual umbrella of self-awareness. This message flows through the book, always present in some way. The key to success is self-awareness, honesty, understanding, and acknowledgement, without judgement, of who we are and where we're going. Just wonderful.

So, let's unpack this message even further.

EI begins with you. The magnificent speaker Jim Rohn, in one of his motivational talks, perfectly applies a metaphor of a flight attendant demonstration before take-off. It's always said during the pre-flight safety briefing that should the aircraft suffer decompression, and the masks drop from the above passenger service unit, you must 'put your mask on first' and only then proceed to help others. So, put your mask on first. This is a textbook metaphor for EI. First get yourself in a good place, then help others. Please refer to Gichin Funakoshi's 20 precepts in your white belt syllabus and check out number 4. It reads, 'First control yourself before attempting to control others'.

In the same way as you can become a student of mindfulness, you can also develop your EI skills. Interestingly, the by-product of this self-mastery is gaining the ability to shine the beacon of attention outwards in the form of empathy, tuning in to others, which is a keystone of EI.

People who are naturally empathetic are blessed as this skill brings out the best in the people around them. They possess a unique way of connecting with people, based on understanding and genuine interest, along with a set of exceptional listening skills.

Yes, empathetic leaders are truly great listeners, who can listen to their own mind, body and spirit on the inside and likewise on the outside they are brilliant at affording others their time and energy. I think we would all agree that when someone gives you their full and present attention it's incredibly empowering and rare. Being made to feel valued and important is the ultimate feeling for any person in a team, organisation or relationship. It is often referred to as psychological safety. And being able to deliver and instil this feeling into others comes after a huge amount of work on yourself.

This is exactly why I inform my clients that when I'm with them, they get the lot! My life, my experience, my skills and my soul. And for that time nothing else exists. Living a black belt life encompasses and embraces EI in such a way that, once it's in place, it becomes deeply embedded and it can be a lifelong skill.

Dr Daniel Goleman breaks this into four parts:
1. **Self-awareness – knowing yourself first**
2. **Self-management – controlling and regulating your emotions**
3. **Empathy – tuning in to others' emotions and perspectives**
4. **Connection/social awareness – the ability to connect with people**

These are all essential elements to black belt leadership and a black belt life. Understanding the fundamentals of our brains, our minds and the relationship between thoughts and feelings, and mind, body and soul will have an immediate and long-lasting impact on your life. It changes you instantaneously and, as I said, it can last forever.

You can do exercises to help you understand, welcome and control your emotions. All you have to do is think about events that have occurred in your past and use them as triggers. Try some exciting experiences, times when you were smiling and laughing and then try some occasions when you were sad. You can gauge your emotional response to these thoughts. Remember, as stated in the yellow belt chapter, the brain doesn't know the difference between real life and illusion.

During my early time in the dojo, I was not skilled in self-awareness and didn't take time out to check in on what I was experiencing. I just battled through. Looking back, one thing I relied on was my inborn 'never give up' mentality. That value of perseverance, which is one of the magical six pillars of the way, runs through this book as a go-to to keep you in check. Never stop using this model as your frame of reference.

My perseverance was pushed to the limit many times. Once I took a short break from karate as it got on top of me both mentally and physically. During my previous grading, when fighting, I had been slipping and sliding in my own blood on the dojo floor through the burst blisters on my feet. I got through and passed but it took away some of that spark. After a few months of not training a really strange thing happened. I think it was an example of synchronicity. My sensei said that he turned and spoke to another sensei about me, just before a training session was about to start. My sensei said, 'I think we've lost him,' meaning me, as it had been months since I had trained, and then I walked through the door of the dojo, bowed and lined up! He looked at me emotionless with his unique, powerful demeanour, and bowed to me, then his face broke into a huge, beaming smile. I was back!

I guess it took some nerve to turn up for my first karate lesson in a pair of Adidas tracksuit bottoms and then do everything that was asked of me incorrectly. Like most of us I suffered hugely from a fear of failure, rejection, humiliation and the unknown. I had a background of success in other sports, so why did I make myself so vulnerable, why did I want to put myself through that test?

As I have said, this book is the result of me unpacking what actually went on in my mind, body and spirit, the challenges I faced, from the desperate feeling of giving up to the euphoria of success; my reactions to my fears and how I dealt with them. I can now see this as an incredible adventure and a reflection of what we face every day in our lives. I've subsequently figured it out and understand exactly what went on inside of me, which puts me in the amazing position of being able to use and share this wisdom to help others including you.

In the white belt syllabus, we began with the mantra 'attitude is everything'. Attitude is a mindset; a way of living. There are many ingredients to living a life of mind and body mastery, a black belt life, but it always starts with our mindset – our thinking. And I'm going to teach you a different way to think about your thoughts! It may sound stupid but bear with me and it will all make sense.

What is the different between mind and thought?

Let's clear up the language. Mind – it's something that produces thought. It's the energy behind thinking. Sydney Banks, a well-known philosopher, author and lecturer said, *'Some believe the brain and mind are two different things, one is biological the other is spiritual.'*

He also said, *'Thought is not reality; yet it is through thought that our realities are created.'* I can't argue with that. Can you?

What happened to me at the start of my journey?

To begin with I went through all the normal emotions relating to doing something new, meeting people for the first time and taking something on that I did not have a clue about. So, what made me do this and want to challenge myself? I had nothing to lose in terms of learning a new skill and philosophy but I must say that those encouraging words from my sensei when I first met him became my new meaning and purpose. They became my inner journey, my *ikigai*. Those words became my secret inner mantra, something everyone should have because it has a profound impact on our thinking.

'Give me twelve months with you and I will get you doing things that you can only dream of!' If that is not inspiration, then I don't know what is and, today, this is exactly how I approach my clients.

What the sensei had given me, in those few words, was inspiration and the promise of adventure which triggered a great deal of motivational neurochemistry.

Bruce Lee said, *'When you find yourself surrounded by enemies you should tell yourself, I am not locked in here with you, you are locked in here with me.'* That kind of mindset will help you succeed in all of your goal-related pursuits.

He had laid down a challenge, a goal with a clear, set in stone process that could lead to outstanding results. On reflection it met with all the GENESIS goal-setting criterion from the red belt syllabus. Wow, this was amazing but was twelve months a short-term goal? I soon found that once I became a part of this perfectly mapped out goal-setting process the goal organically moved to the longer term and then into a way of life.

Originally, the truth was that the goal of becoming a black belt was not real to me. It was too far away so I couldn't imagine it, I couldn't find those necessary mental pictures. Initially, I just couldn't believe it, which is a critical element in achieving success. You must have belief. As much as I tried, I could not get my imagination to sketch out the black belt around my waist. I couldn't even faintly conceive it to start with and, at times, it seemed impossible.

The beauty of this process, however, was the visibility of the clear strategy of small steps to achieve the goal, along with timelines, milestones and check-ins. The bulletproof process and structure for measurement of progress was already in place for me. The configuration was already there, all I had to do was turn up with the right attitude and learn to adhere and respect the precepts and culture. A cliché maybe, but I took it one session at a time, one belt at a time, but always with the right attitude, knowing I was on a journey. This is exactly how you should approach change.

We covered goal setting as a red belt and what a magnificent process this was, with all the coloured belts to measure exactly where you are positioned in the process. Each belt cleverly provides you with a standing of achievement and the next colour challenges you to learn more, develop your skills, emotions and mindset. Think about it, I only needed to look to my right and there was the next step to my goal, wrapped around a student's waist. Orange, red, yellow and so on. There was my picture, I didn't need to imagine it, it was literally right next to me in real time. This is how a goal-setting process should be and I have proven that it can be achieved outside of the dojo.

This entire procedure became the inspiration behind my coaching practice and, subsequently, this book. I now successfully demonstrate my own system, which helps others firstly discover, and then unlock, their potential, their inner belts. That is precisely what I do professionally.

So, life in the dojo became my metaphor for the inner world. Our mind is our dojo and, at times, we need to bow and enter it in a spiritual not

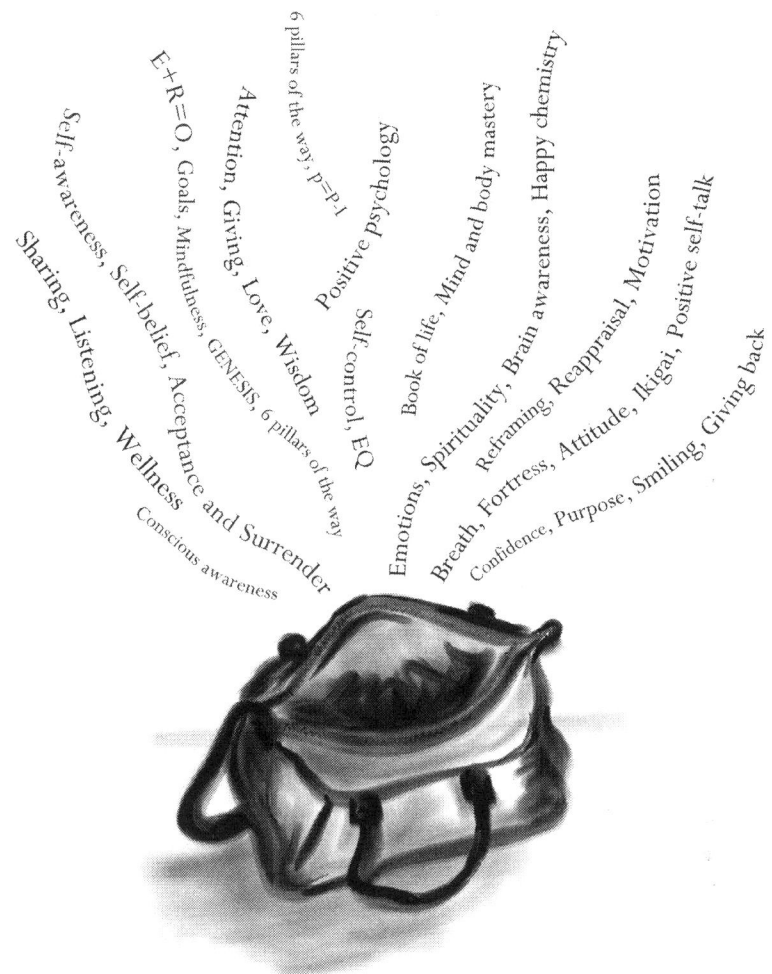

physical way. I guarantee this is the secret to living a black belt life.

So, as with karate, we set out inspirational goals, then formulate a process to reach them. With the measurement of progress cleverly mapped out with smaller landmark rewards along the way – it delivers vision, an indestructible plan and both clarity and certainty to satisfy our needy brains with the bonus requirement in the form of adventure. Remember the paradox of certainty – we need both the known to keep us present and to explore the unknown to help us grow.

However, that said, we know nothing can be achieved without the right attitude, and this is driven home from day one in the dojo (and the beginning of this book). The right attitude has within it a willingness, respect, belief, positivity and perseverance that will supply you with everything you are searching for. You have heard the saying 'seek and you shall find'. Unless you search you will discover nothing.

Before we enter the grading exam, let's recap on what has emerged in our brains, our minds, our bodies, our emotions and our spirit.

We heard that skills and knowledge are critical in performance but what takes you to success, whatever success looks like, is your state of mind. It's your attitude that will get you over the line. The power of the mind is astonishing and, therefore, committing to understanding it and respecting it is a game changer in respect of your learning.

In controlling our emotions, we looked at anger being the enemy. We can use the two formulas covered in this book, E+R=O and p=P-I, to help us. The first is to determine what response is needed to achieve any desired outcome and the next is making sure that we move out of the way of ourselves to fast track to growth and achievement.

From day one of the journey, it was said we live in two worlds; an inner world of self-awareness, self-reflection, self-regulation and continuous development and an outer world of external factors not in our control that we find challenging us every day. By following the journey of the book, maintaining the inside-out living philosophy, learning and flourishing, doing the drills, creating new exciting habits, constantly working on your identity – your self-version and filling your kitbag with various tools then our life becomes one world. Our perspective shifts to a world of opportunity and abundance, a world of love, wisdom and growth, a world of mindfulness, gratefulness and a world that also helps others on their journey.

To conclude this adventure, I want to end by sharing with you what happens after the actual grading to black belt. I was awarded a beautiful silk belt by my club. It was made in Japan and had my name on one end and the name of the institution I trained under on the other, all in Japanese. Over time, the black silk wears away, as you can see on the cover of this book, and the belt actually turns white. How remarkable it is to see this and let me tell you why... For me it symbolises the circle of life. We start as a white belt; we get to black and then, over time, go back to white. It's like we are starting all over again. In fact, we are doing exactly that. Never stopping, always moving forward. Isn't that just beautiful.

In the dojo, we are taught not to stop or slow down our learning and development, to always keep moving forward; it is a culture of transcendence. If you check back to the white belt syllabus and Gichin Funakoshi's twenty precepts, the eleventh is 'Karate is like boiling water. If you do not heat it constantly it will cool'.

This entire chapter, the black belt syllabus, is essentially and intentionally the warm-up to your black belt grading. It has delivered to you the opportunity to truly dial in and reflect on your journey to this very moment. Its purpose is to help you revisit your own unique and personal adventure of learning and self-discovery, capturing your findings when unlocking those chambers of inner treasures. But also to return you to your breakthroughs, those special and insightful 'aha' moments you have experienced along the way. And, finally, to review and revise the drills, tools and wisdom you have acquired to help others on their pathways. You are now prepared for your black belt grading.

You are so close…you just need to complete the final test.

Good luck.

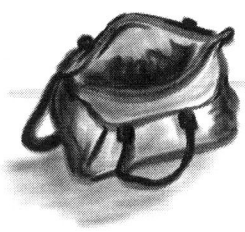

BLACK BELT GRADING

1. As with the circle of life, turn back time to a white belt, then orange and revisit your values and belief structure, your fortress. Make any adjustments and lock them down as they will be navigating you to your new and life-changing goal-bound destinations.
2. Describe what changes you are going to implement. What exactly are your true goals? Use GENESIS and then apply to the process the six pillars of the way to guarantee your success.
3. Write down the three key takeaways from each syllabus for you. Have you experienced any transformational learning and development from this experience? Describe the impact.
4. Revisit and define your meaning and purpose, your fuel that drives you forward. This is your *ikigai.*
5. Describe in your own unique style what living a black belt life means to you.
6. Note how your amazing feat of self-discovery can materialise into helping and supporting others.
7. Could you become a black belt leader? What changes do you need to make?
8. Finally, and most importantly, the question most used in coaching: what next for you?

'If you can dream it, you can do it.' ~ WALT DISNEY

You've done it!
Congratulations, my kind readers.
You have become a black belt.
Now it's time to live a black belt life.

'A black belt is a white belt who never quits.' ~ RENZO GRACIE

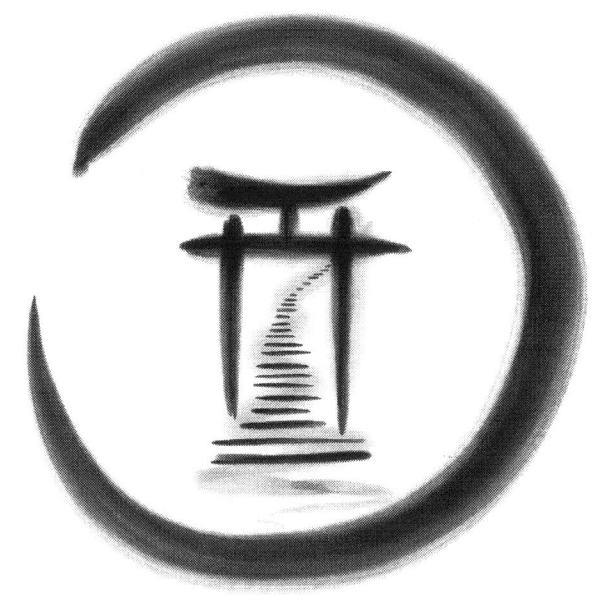

CHAPTER 9
BEYOND BLACK BELT

'You are never too old to set another goal or to dream a new dream.' ~ C.S. LEWIS

In martial arts, once you become a black belt you are a black belt forever. But what happens once you achieve your goal? As I discovered, becoming a black belt is actually the starting point not the finish line.

It's said in martial arts that when you become a black belt that's when you start to learn. This is so true. Reaching a goal for me is reaching a gateway of life. A gateway to step through into a new way of living. It's not the end, it's the beginning. It's the starting line.

As a coach I tend to use running a marathon for the first time as a pretty accurate metaphor to unpack what steps are needed in a seriously challenging process. There are many stages, as you can imagine. What I point out, though, is the process, the way, that takes you to the start line, not the finish. This is key, the goal is there to be reached but you cannot stop, you must keep moving. I see my clients smash through their goals and continue on to achieve wonderful things. It's incredible to witness.

Now you have reached this level of awareness it's about a shift in dynamic.

One day I asked my sensei, 'What is the meaning and purpose of our roles as sensei?'

He said, 'To pass on our knowledge and skills to others' and repeated a Zen proverb. 'When the student is ready the teacher appears. That's it, this is what we were born to do.'

Therefore, earning this belt brings with it a responsibility. A responsibility to share your experiences, challenges and successes with others. You will be able to conduct yourself in a different way, a way that symbolises your accomplishments, which infiltrate all four aspects of life – mental, physical, spiritual and emotional. Leading yourself first, for me, is fundamental for all great leaders.

As you experience the transformation from brown to black belt a sense of leadership naturally manifests. I experienced it first-hand. Something changed, something emotional, and possibly spiritual. I immediately felt the need to help others and pass on my knowledge.

Even now, when donning the black belt, it still feels like something special occurs, every single time. However, strangely, it's not karate itself and the skills I developed that come to mind, it's the feeling of respect and accomplishment. Respect for the way, respect for what the journey teaches you and respect for reaching a new understanding of yourself. When you wrap the black belt around your waist you are taken to another gateway, which opens to a never-ending path to self-mastery – always learning and moving, but this time, forever sharing; helping others find their own way to living a black belt life.

The Buddha said: 'Thousands of candles can be lighted from a single candle, and the life of the candle will not be shortened. Happiness never decreases by being shared.' I want this book to be the flame that lights many candles. I truly believe you all can find the way, whatever that looks like for you and however you want to design it. It's in there waiting for you. It's in front of you. You have the capability to create change in so many different ways that will positively affect your life and those of others.

This is what successful karate students do, they learn something new, work hard to master it and move on to learn something else, always pushing beyond their comfort zone and constantly developing new skills and ways of understanding.

I feel it is vitally important to mention that, as a part of their continuous improvement ethos and attention to detail, black belts spend a great deal of time going back to the core basics of their martial art to see if they can notice something they missed, discover something new or apply what they have learned in a different way.

They return to the other area of the dojo where they teach white belts, at the beginning of their journey, the basics and the precepts. This process also helps black belts to continue to refine their own skills and techniques, to benefit from the learning of others. And it is critical for you to adopt this attitude.

The most beautiful thing about all black belts, all senseis, is that they started as a white belt, every single one of them. And this brings with it a unique connection to their students, the mutual respect, empathy and appreciation of the challenges and rewards ahead. And you can also take this lead outside the dojo into the world of business, sport and other environments.

There is a great quote by John C. Maxwell, a New York bestselling author, coach and speaker that says, 'A leader is one who knows the way, goes the way, and shows the way.'

In my mind a black belt leader helps you find the way.

Black belt leadership is about an understanding. How do you get the best out of others, what makes people tick, what makes people perform as individuals and then as a team? How do you inspire others to go on to become black belt leaders in their own right? When you have the answers, the wisdom and you have walked the way, you can call yourself a sensei.

In my lifetime I have learnt so much through various pursuits but nothing more so than the importance of being a team player. Personally, I love to learn and absorb all I can from any situation and then, most importantly, share want I've learned so others can benefit.

There is a point when we are no longer the receiver, but the transmitter. When we stop following and take the lead.

Watching, listening and learning from other senseis of life is central to success. We all know who they are. They are personal to us and from all walks of life. Family, friends, colleagues; true role models. Most of us will come into contact with just a few people in our lives that leave a lifelong positive impression. This unique group are our private influencers, they are our signposts, the guides that give us direction and inspiration and the encouragement for us to grow.

It is said we can always recall certain people in our lives, those who either changed us or had a profound impact on our direction, personality or behaviour. These people are like demigods, they have a special presence, something different, something outstanding, something you want desperately to have yourself. Consequently, we mould ourselves on these wonderful human beings, and I acknowledge some of the important people who have influenced my life at the end of this book.

In truth I still learn from everyone. I love to watch and listen to people, more now than ever before and I am constantly inspired by my clients. They are now my teachers.

And then, of course, there is my sensei, Peter. He is quite extraordinary. If you made a list of twenty values, he would have them all in some form. He is eighty-eight as I write and still dons his gi and black belt with pride. He has lived a remarkable life and, although he is the strongest person I have ever met, in so many ways, he is also humble and always, without fail, there for you. The day I met him changed my life forever. He possesses a presence, an aura that few have, that I found so intriguing. When he walks into a room, not just a dojo, you feel it. It's something beyond normality.

When teaching in the dojo it used to baffle me how he appeared to see everything that was going on. He had a sixth sense or a human radar that locked in on anyone that wasn't pulling their weight. To receive a nod of acknowledgement from him felt like you'd won the lottery. It produced a massive shot of dopamine.

None of his students can believe how he has maintained his core strength, posture, control and technique well into his eighties. You felt proud when he pulled you out of the line to demonstrate various moves using you as the crash test dummy.

I was pulled out many times, but I remember one episode in particular, when he was explaining to the class how to achieve serious distance and execute a devastating blow to someone. One thing about me was that I never flinched and never moved when an attack was being demonstrated on me. I trusted my senseis, well most of them. However, on this occasion, my sensei's control was 1% out as his hammer fist demonstration thudded into my chest. Six weeks later I was back training again after my ribs had repaired! I sometimes wish it had left a scar as sort of a badge of honour, because, strangely, I'm quite proud of receiving that blow.

With all that power and presence, along with my mum, he is the most empathetic, attentive and understanding listener I have ever been in the company of. Reflect for a minute or two and think about who your life senseis have been to this point…this is part of your journey.

Now I'd like to share a story about Winston Churchill's mother, Jennie Jerome, who had separate dinners with William Gladstone and Benjamin Disraeli a week before the election, around the mid-19th century. A journalist asked Jennie what her impression of the two men was. She responded, 'When I left the dining room after being with Gladstone, I thought he was the most interesting man in England. But when I left the dining room after being with Disraeli, I felt like I was the most interesting woman in England.'

Disraeli had mastered the art of listening and making other people feel respected and important, a secret ingredient to being a great leader and human being. Guess who won the election – yes, Benjamin Disraeli!

They say great leaders are both interested and interesting, I think that's a perfect way to describe a black belt leader and even more appropriate for Sensei Peter. After my black belt grading, I gave him a gift, with a note sincerely thanking him for all his support and guidance and for sharing his deep and widespread wisdom to get me there. His response was a note saying, 'I didn't do it, you did! All I did was open the door for you and you went through it like a bolt of lightning.' And this is exactly how I see my practice of coaching.

Self-awareness
Has clarity
Emotionally intelligent
Ethical
A great listener
Empathic
Courageous
Confident
Possesses integrity
Wise
Present
Resilient
Kind
Compassionate
Inspirational
Passionate
A role model
Has humility
Coaches
Has faith
Self-belief
Enchanting
Extracts the best from people
Has a sense of humour
Respectful and respected
Knowledgeable
Communicates
Possesses a keen eye for detail
Accountable
Engaged
Loyal

And this is how I want you, my kind and incredible readers, to see this book. As a doorway, as the gateway to wonderful things and for all of you to go through it like a bolt of lightning.

Like all great senseis, great leaders have a set of very special qualities. They communicate in a way that makes you feel special and important, they make you feel that anything is possible.

From those people who have inspired and influenced me in some way, let's draw on some key strengths and values they possess and see where it takes us.

It's no coincidence that the illustration on the previous page represents what amazing leaders have at their disposal – what they have in their own personal kitbags. Remember, great leaders lead themselves first.

WHAT IS 'LIVING A BLACK BELT LIFE'?

It's a state of mind that I assure you any one of us can live with. I have lived a black belt for many years now and my life has been transformed. Today, I understand what it took to reach that level in terms of the psychology and physiology made up from the quadrant of life – my physical, mental, emotional and spiritual strength and development. It was monumental.

My dojo adventure was a more extreme, violent and physically demanding, but equally powerful, version of the bamboo tree fable in the white belt syllabus. I suffered blistered and bleeding feet for years, and, as described, would sometimes slip and slide in my own blood. I suffered many cracked ribs, black eyes, cuts, bruises and a damaged eye socket. Let me add snapped ankle ligaments, torn hamstrings and groin, chronic tendonitis and a plethora of other muscle injuries. But I just kept going back, every week, every month, every year, as did the bamboo tree gardener. The day I became a black belt I felt like the bamboo tree that shoots up 90 feet in just a few weeks after years of nurturing, but my realisation of achievement shot 90 feet the moment that the sensei announced it. It was simply the best feeling I have ever experienced.

My black belt life has helped me to discover who my best friend is. It's me. It took many decades to eventually find and meet him and one of the fundamental objectives of this book is to help you see that there is no need to go as long as I did to find your best friend.

A black belt life becomes a superpower as a result of all the challenges, successes, adversity and failures we have faced and come through. The power has been earned through a life of continuous growth and raising standards. Always evolving, practising new skills, new ways to think while developing your strengths, unlocking your potential and harnessing them to deliver magnificent results. And yes, for sure, it all starts with the awareness of self. It's living life from the inside out.

This attitude of life gives you a sense of freedom; freedom from self-criticism and low self-worth. At the same time, you gain feelings of optimism, honesty and acceptance. The freedom to constantly explore the inner self and the liberating acceptance of your strengths and weaknesses as a human being. It translates as expressing a deep sense of gratitude which, as we covered along the way, is essentially the main ingredient of happiness.

A black belt life provides you with a spiritual presence, a burning glow of self-belief and confidence which allows you to dream big and set out plans to achieve life-changing goals.

It's having a life containing mindfulness, spending much time in the present moment while removing blame and judgement from the 'R' in our E+R=O formula. It's enabling you to become 'the listener', a brilliant listener, firstly paying close attention to your mind and body, then directing your skills and attention to helping others.

A black belt life delivers an incredible feeling of passion, clarity and control and a special meaning and purpose that gets us up, dialled in and alive and kicking every day. A black belt life.

I cannot express how sincere I am when I say I hope *You Can Live a Black Belt Life* has been more than a self-help and personal development book. I hope you have found moments of inspiration and discovery and you feel you have been on an adventure of self-exploration. I truly hope it's been transformational for you.

'If you always put limits on everything you do, physical or anything else, it will spread into your work and into your life. There are no limits. There are only plateaus, and you must not stay there, you must go beyond them.' ~ BRUCE LEE

ACKNOWLEDGEMENTS

Firstly, I'd like to acknowledge those who have influenced me as a person during the course of my life. Many have played a small part in my life movie but the main characters, my movie stars, are but a few.

MY MUM, SHIRLEY – a war evacuee, taken from her parents living in London during the Second World War. Someone who struggled with confidence all her life but is, without question, the kindest person and best listener I have ever known.

MY FATHER, EDDIE – a small man in height but captured within his frame is a resilience to behold. Living with and battling Parkinson's disease for many years, beating cancer, he is ninety-one years old and still going as I write this book.

MY WIFE, DONNA – whom I met nearly forty years ago, has supported me through thick and thin. A tremendously loyal, hardworking person who has faced, and dealt with, her own life challenges in a way that is an inspiration to me and others. Thank you for being there.

MY DAUGHTER, ELLIE – when she gets within a hundred feet of me my face lights up. She has become more than a daughter; she has become a devoted friend, too. Someone I love spending time with and someone I draw my life energy from.

MY SENSEI PETER – to whom I owe a debt of gratitude. That moment, that chance meeting altered my course of life. He could see things about me that I couldn't and set about taking me on an adventure to a place where anything is possible.

STUART S – my brother-in-law who, over the years, has become the brother I never had. I just love being in his company. From me being his biggest fan, watching him evolve from an eleven-year-old into an elite footballer, he has become one of my greatest supporters.

PETER – a close friend and true gentleman whom I met at the age of twenty-two when I moved cricket clubs. He took me under his wing and became a great friend. Sadly, he is no longer with us but rarely a week goes by where I do not think of him. At the packed service of his passing his son David gave a beautiful and touching eulogy during which he said that many people described his father as someone who, whether you met him for one minute or one hour, you felt better about life when you walked away. What a legacy!

ADRIAN – my mindfulness teacher. It's said that some things are meant to happen. Meeting him was one of those special moments never to be forgotten. In that brief first meeting my life changed forever. My gratitude for that moment and the many times we met thereafter is unsurpassed. His incredible method of teaching is actually not teaching, it's guiding you to a wisdom that cannot be challenged, only learned, understood and translated into your own language.

RICHARD – a close and true friend and former teammate, who was a fierce competitor on the cricket field and became a globally successful, first-class, internationally recognised cricket coach. He is the one that encouraged me to take up life and performance coaching professionally. I cannot thank him enough for his persistence and confidence in me.

JANE – another great friend and successful executive coach. A while ago, while having a coffee together in London I asked her what I should do to enhance my coaching life and practice. She said, 'You need to write a book. You have a great story to tell.' Well, Jane, I've done it!

DAVID TS WOOD – a schoolmate who after leaving school we met up again. The thing was it was after forty years! Now living in BC Canada and a hugely successful businessman, motivational speaker and coach, we have become great friends and he too is a constant driver and inspiration to me.

STUART B – they say everyone has one person they could and would call if they were in serious trouble and were desperate for help. This is the person I would call because I know he would pick up the phone. A former captain of mine he is a wonderful friend whom I have had the pleasure to know for almost forty years.

TIM – another friend stretching over many decades. He said he was inspired by my leadership on the field of play when we played cricket together. He went on to become hugely successful in the City of London and is a wonderful human being. He is another who encouraged me to help others through my coaching skills. Thank you for your support, Tim.

MIKE – with whom I have a loyal and trusted friendship, spanning nearly four decades.

BEN – a devoted and supportive friend, client and business partner.

AMY – my wonderful copywriter and loyal pillar of support and encouragement who has been with me through the entire process of writing this book. Her energy and enthusiasm would light up any room and it's been a pleasure to work with her.

KIM – my brilliant editor who has not just skilfully edited my book, never detracting from my writing style and message, but also taken time out to introduce and educate me in a new world of becoming an author. I'm looking forward to working with Kim on my next book.

LEO – my illustrator. Thank you for your amazing illustrations throughout the book. They are genius.

BARRY – my cover designer and formatter. It's been a pleasure working with you and to experience and appreciate your incredible craft and creativity.

All the wonderful friends that came from school, work, on the cricket field and football pitch, in the gym and the dojo, and on my travels.

A very special place – The Swan at Lavenham, Suffolk. This beautiful, oak-beamed hotel, based in the historic village of Lavenham, is where a great many of my client meetings take place. It holds a unique presence and energy, a feeling of warmth and welcome creating an environment which I found to be conducive to my coaching sessions. Many clients have experienced transformational shifts to their lives there and often find themselves returning to the hotel to stay or dine in celebration of life.

My place of the way, my dojo – Stoke by Nayland resort, Essex. The place I met Sensei Peter and my life changed forever. We still train there twenty years on.

Lastly, but by no means least, my clients who never fail to amaze me with their own personal stories of adversity, their honesty and their dreams. To witness such commitment to create a new life, digging deep to find the strength and determination to succeed on their, sometimes challenging but always insightful, unique adventures of self-discovery and transformation is a joy and, at times, breathtakingly rewarding. They are a constant and reliable source of utter inspiration.

MY VIRTUAL MOTIVATIONAL MENTORS:

Jim Rohn
Tony Robins
Jack Canfield
Wayne Dyer
Bob Proctor
Les Brown
Sydney Banks
Zig Ziglar

AUTHORS OF INFLUENCE:

Dr David Rock
Urban Myer
James Clear
Mihaly Csikszentmihalyi
Allen Carr
Don Miguel Ruiz
Dr Carol S Dweck
Michael Neill
Eckhart Tolle
John Kabat-Zin
Ken Mogi
Daniel Goleman

ABOUT THE AUTHOR

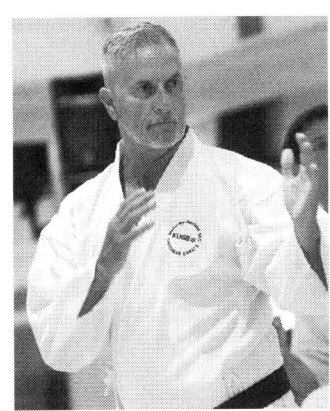

Phil is a successful life and transformational coach.

Throughout his life he has shown an unrelenting love of sport, fitness and well-being, martial arts, leadership and, above all, personal development. He has also been a passionate student of mindfulness for many years.

He trained with the NeuroLeadership Institute, becoming a brain-based coach, and has since continued with his quest for knowledge, studying positive psychology and well-being, neuroscience and emotional intelligence, all supporting his mission in helping people to grow or transform. He has taken this, together with his own work/life experiences, a lifetime in team sports, and the proven principles of karate, to create his own unique, powerful and successful coaching system that has subsequently delivered incredible results.

Born in Sudbury, Suffolk, Phil now resides in the historic village of Lavenham where the streets and houses were famously used for scenes in the Harry Potter movie franchise.

Printed in Poland
by Amazon Fulfillment
Poland Sp. z o.o., Wrocław
03 October 2022

4133a83b-9e66-43fb-850e-a29a4a420935R01